IMAGINING CRIMINOLOGY

AN ALTERNATIVE PARADIGM

FRANK P. WILLIAMS III

T0352722

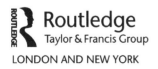
Routledge
Taylor & Francis Group

LONDON AND NEW YORK

First published 1999 by Garland Publishing, Inc.

2 Park Square, Milton Park, Abingdon, Oxfordshire OX14 4RN
52 Vanderbilt Avenue, New York, NY 10017

Routledge is an imprint of the Taylor & Francis Group, an informa business

First issued in paperback 2019

Library of Congress Cataloging-in-Publication Data

Williams, Franklin P.
   Imagining criminology : an alternative paradigm / by Frank P.
Williams III.
      p.   cm. — (Garland reference library of social science ; v. 1183.
Current issues in criminal justice ; v. 24)
      Includes bibliographical references and index.
      ISBN 0-8153-3078-2 (alk. paper)
      1. Criminology—Philosophy.   I. Title.   II. Series: Garland reference
library of social science ; v. 1183.   III. Series: Garland reference library of
social science. Current issues in criminal justice ; v. 24.
   HV6018.W49   1999
   364—dc21   98-42229
                                                                          CIP

ISBN 13: 978-0-8153-3078-3 (hbk)
ISBN 13: 978-1-138-88032-0 (pbk)

IMAGINING
CRIMINOLOGY

CURRENT ISSUES IN CRIMINAL JUSTICE
VOLUME 24
GARLAND REFERENCE LIBRARY OF SOCIAL SCIENCE
VOLUME 1183

To Marilyn McShane, my mate and best friend

Contents

Series Editor's Foreword

As we conclude our work on the series Current Issues in Criminal Justice, I am very proud that the last contribution is *Imagining Criminology*. The book represents another milestone in a criminologist's journey to uncover some "truths" about the discipline and to reflect critically on how that field has evolved. This journey, some of you may remember, began in *The Sociology of Criminological Theory: Paradigm or Fad* and continued in *The Demise of the Criminological Imagination*. To date, this latest work has already attracted considerable debate and in the tradition of C. Wright Mills, engendered somewhat heated discussion about the philosophy of criminology and the logic of its paradigms. What is perhaps most exciting about this work is that it is critical, in the true sense of critical, a term that has been abused and overused.

As editor, partner, and colleague of Frank Williams, it has been exciting to watch *Imagining Criminology* unfold, in a series of papers, and late night beer drinking discussions, hours on the computer staring at chaos models and sitting on the beach watching the ocean. Although the reader may not always agree about the state of the art of criminology, he or she will enjoy thinking through this book. It is an exercise in professional self-examination and it is a good workout.

Marilyn D. McShane

Preface

Most authors tend to leave readers in the dark over the assumptions they make and the way in which they come to the ideas of the work. Because I believe these are important pieces in understanding what someone has to say, this preface is oriented toward making these pieces explicit. Thus, readers will find a personal odyssey and acknowledgments in these pages—all designed to show how this book came to be and the influences that created it.

The idea for this book had its genesis over the past two decades. It seemed to me the approaches taken by various criminological theories were somewhat isolated. Each theory was seen as something different and each had its own set of champions. Rarely was anyone interested in combining and integrating theories; when it did happen, the effort seemed to interest very few. In one sense, this was surprising. The major theorists of the 1950s (Cohen, Cloward and Ohlin) were integrators, combining the Chicago School and anomie traditions. Therefore, two questions bothered me. What had we lost in the 1970s and 1980s? Why weren't these separate theories seen as alternative and complementary views of reality rather than right and wrong views?

Another question should have bothered me as well: why was I asking these questions when no one else was? In retrospect, this last question was probably the easiest to answer. I came from a different background than most criminologists, being only nominally the product of a sociology education. My undergraduate education contained as much coursework in the natural sciences as the social sciences. I did brief graduate coursework in public administration and traffic engineering before deciding on criminology, and the latter choice was not then a product of actually knowing and liking criminology.

Graduate education at Florida State was also a bit different than most sociological criminologists experienced. First, we were not in sociology, but were a separate school of criminology. Second, two people there were doing different sorts of things for the criminology of that period. Ron Akers was developing his social learning theory and graduate students were getting heavy doses of operant psychology. C. Ray Jeffery was duplicating the infusion of operant psychology and then lecturing on environmental design and psycho-socio-biology. The graduate students, at least the small group of which I was a part, loved to take these theoretical ideas and discuss them (and there was many a good-natured argument). Most of them, however, seemed to focus on the sociological aspects of theory. That struck me, then and now, as only looking at one part of the explanatory puzzle. Where was the psychology? The biology? The physical environment?

As a result of this feeling, I probably got along with, and spent more time with, C. Ray Jeffery than the rest of my graduate cohort. Meanwhile, Ron Akers, who became my mentor, was encouraging students to investigate all manner of theoretical concepts. One of the things he said that stuck in my mind was that he did not believe that we should follow in his footsteps and become social learning theorists. But for that comment, I probably would have done just that. Instead, I made a concerted effort to do other things.

Another major influence on this book was my reading of Thomas Kuhn's *The Structure of Scientific Revolutions*. It seemed to me that his philosophical history of the natural sciences was right-on. Further, my natural science background led me to believe that most sociologists were reading too much into Kuhn's work. His paradigms were not the wholesale world assumptions they saw. He was talking about the way in which small groups of highly specialized scientists came to an issue with the same problem-solving approach. Of course, it made sense that sociologists saw the meta-picture every time they talked about paradigms. Thus, I originally argued against the presence of paradigms in criminology. In the strict Kuhnian sense I still do, but now at least the overpowering presence of quantitative methodology leads me to believe in an overarching meta-paradigm. And, in that larger sense, I came to believe that mainstream criminology (and most of the social sciences) was (and is) viewing reality from a very narrow perspective.

How could this perspective be enlarged? That is where my first readings of chaos theory came into play. Like most occasional dabblers in the literature of the natural sciences, Gleick's best-selling 1987 book on chaos was my introduction. This seemed to be a good method for enlarging perspectives of reality, but there was no appropriate way I could find to translate chaos theory in criminology (although others certainly tried: see Pepinsky, 1991; Young, 1991). Then, I ran across a copy of *Nature* with an article by Per Bak and colleagues on a chaos-theory offshoot they had developed. That approach, called self-organized criticality theory, provided the idea I had been seeking for using chaos theory. Thus, I began playing with the idea of a non-linear accumulation of factors and a chaotic precipitating incident for behavior. An initial foray into the concepts led to a paper written for the 1990 meeting of the American Society of Criminology. However, I was not comfortable with the approach at that point, which had been mostly conceived as unit theory.

The rest fell gradually into place as I was forced to think more about the meaning of a non-linear critical-incident. Perhaps the most important precipitating event was an invitation by Jeff Walker to be the "guest lecturer" for one of the final weeks in his spring semester, 1994, list-server-based graduate theory class. He was interested in something new and "postmodern." Asked if chaos theory would fit, he agreed and I began writing a very strange first version of critical-incident metatheory. The students of that class were receptive and had many questions about the approach. In answering their questions and responding to queries from Jeff and others who had "taught" a week and were still hanging on (Mike Lynch and Hal Pepinsky), I clarified a number of concepts with which I had been struggling. Two years of intermittent work after that point led to the draft manuscript behind this book and a preliminary version of the metatheory published in *Social Pathology*.

Acknowledgments

As is the usual case, I am indebted to countless people for getting me to this point. Discussions with many colleagues and friends over the years provided various ideas that have been incorporated into the book, and I wish to thank them. At the risk of affronting some by omitting their names, those I can remember in specific conversations, are, in no particular order, Marilyn McShane, Les Wilkins, Sy Dinitz, Ron Akers, C. Ray Jeffery, Frank Scarpitti, Al Reiss, Jeff Ferrell, Jeff Walker, Pete Kraska, Dennis Longmire, Vic Kappeler, Gil Geis, Hal Pepinsky, Austin Turk, Mark Hamm, Lisa Callahan, David Gulick, Mike Lynch, Carl Wagoner, David Shichor, Dale Sechrest, Mickey Braswell, Bob Bohm, Sam Souryal, Mike Blankenship, Kate Jamieson, Vic Strecher, Frank Cullen, Chuck Fields, Mary Parker and Rolando del Carmen. Of those, I wish to acknowledge a major debt to Gil Geis, Jeff Walker, Jeff Ferrell, Mickey Braswell, and Austin Turk, all of whom read and commented on various portions of the manuscript. What is more, they even encouraged me to continue writing it. In addition, I wish to tell all of my old students (and there are a large number of them) that I learned more from them than they ever did from me. I deeply appreciate their patience while I fumbled through the rudimentary ideas of the manuscript and their insights when they saw things more clearly than I did. As is usual under such circumstances, I absolve all of my colleagues and friends from the burden of being associated with such strangeness. I alone am guilty of taking their ideas and making less of them than they could.

I should also acknowledge my editor (and friend) David Estrin at Garland Publishing. David had the foresight to agree that this book would not, by itself, ruin the sterling reputation built over Garland's decades of publishing scholarly works. He also contributed innumerable humorous anecdotes that made me laugh when I was in danger of taking myself too seriously. Phyllis Korper did her usual excellent job of proofing the manuscript and making sure that it was reasonably intelligible.

Finally, there is one person to whom I am indebted beyond description: my "spousal unit," Marilyn McShane. She supported my efforts, gave me ideas, sporadically castigated me when I needed it, and read and edited the draft manuscript. She even graciously suffered the heat and Santa Ana winds of Southern California while I walked the cliffs and beaches of the central California coast on an idyllic sabbatical where most of the chapters of the book were written. I appreciate her in more ways than she will ever understand.

It now remains to be seen if the materials to follow justify Marilyn's faith in me or, in one of her favorite sayings, help to fill a much needed gap in the literature.

Imagining
Criminology

CHAPTER ONE

Thought and Ideology

INTRODUCTION

This book is a product of a growing unease about the criminological enterprise. And it is not solely my unease, because I have heard many colleagues express similar opinions in discussions at conferences and meetings. Nor is this feeling a new one; it began for me in the early 1980s. The essence of the problem seems to be a perception that we have been doing the same thing for a long time and have little to show for it. At the very least, there is a foreboding that we have reached a point of diminishing returns (Charles Wellford [1989], for instance, talks about a state of "theoretical paralysis."). I know that many criminologists will disagree with these statements and reply that we have progressed greatly. While that may be true—and, clearly, that is a matter of perspective—I think it is only true over the longer time span of this century. The proper question is whether we are progressing much at this point. More than disagreeing with the commentary (or pieces of it) in this book, some will be appalled with the thrust of the argument. Those people, I expect, will be those whose careers (or training) have been vested in current empirical methodology and positivistic theory construction. In part, that is exactly what I wish to challenge. Others will object to the "discursive" form of theorizing (Gibbons, 1994) in the latter chapters. Because I intend to propose a metatheory, rather than a unit theory, there are no specific empirical hypotheses to be made. I will make an effort, however, to posit relationships with existing unit theories and ferret out some possible empirical points of examination. In the end, though, the style will remain discursive.

THE DIFFICULTY OF THINKING

I simply don't believe we are devoting much time to *thinking*. Very few graduate students over the past 20 years have had courses in logic and almost none have explored materials in the broad subject areas of creativity. The move toward specialization has likewise had a deleterious effect on thinking. Few scholars take time to explore issues beyond their specialization and, even when they do, the exploration is likely to be constrained by their disciplinary identity (i.e., thinking only *within* one's discipline). Moreover, the chase for objectivity and rigor in contemporary work has caused us to lose an appreciation for the essential richness of human behavior. On the whole, criminological scholars have become rather shortsighted.[1]

The Emphasis on Empiricism

Social scientists (and scientists in general) partake of certain assumptions about the proper way to conceive of the universe, yet most scientists are not particularly aware of them. Such unawareness is not surprising because world assumptions (Gouldner, 1970) are not normally expressed and constitute the background against which our most profound belief systems operate. These assumptions (generality, determinism, parsimony and empiricism) create a world view of a universe that is purposive and observable. Though all four of these assumptions affect the way in which knowledge is pursued and attained, two of them—parsimony and generality—have special import for criminology. By uncritically accepting parsimony and generality, research and theory have undertaken to reduce the complexity of life to as few variables as possible. Moreover, the *social* sciences generally prefer that those significant variables are found in the greatest number of people. The end product is a form of reductionism: understanding of complexity is best achieved through simplicity. In short, the search for understanding has been reduced to a more modest task—explanation—which requires no intrinsic depth. And we have failed even that, as judged by empirical evidence for our explanations.

But I do not reject positivistic empirical methodology: I simply think it unwise to rely on any single methodology to the extent the social sciences do now. While I believe that such work has been constructive, I also believe we now must overcome a strict reliance on it and get on with understanding people. This view is certainly not unique. C. Wright Mills in *The Sociological Imagination* noted that sociologists of the 1950s had already engaged in the pursuit of too much empiricism and too little theory. Furthermore, it is a virtual certainty that all modern criminologists are aware of that classic work. It is ironic, then, that anyone should need to discuss the dangers of overemphasizing empiricism. Yet it seems that we have largely ignored Mills' (1959:6) message: one needs "to grasp history and biography and the relations between the two with society" to understand current social realities. A half century later, it is time to take the criticism to heart. We need to pursue imagination as one way of understanding reality and that is done by understanding the context of social phenomena. Mills also said (1959:4) that ordinary men do not possess the quality of mind to grasp the interplay of larger issues on the lives of people. Thus, we must turn to those chosen to pursue graduate work in the social sciences—those who are, or should be, trained to have that quality of mind. This makes it doubly imperative that those people actually use that quality of mind. A failure to do so is partially a waste of training and more broadly a loss for society.

Why should we pursue imagination now? An overweening emphasis on technique and empiricism has done more than simply decrease our sense of the real world. The raw empiricism of much of today's published literature is producing a wealth of articles that are atheoretical, use poor data, are conceptually inadequate, and statistically indefensible. In short, the articles are meaningless to others and picayune; they do not contribute to knowledge. So why are they published? Most likely the answer is that research and publication must be done for tenure and promotion. If that is so, then a major turnabout has occurred: journals now exist to perpetuate the field and the people in it. Articles are frequently published because academics pursue survival, not necessarily because there is anything worth saying. Those who have served on tenure and promotion committees and acted as manuscript reviewers can testify that this is not far from the truth.

The Mode of Education

In addition to the empiricism problem, I believe we have exacerbated our lack of imagination through educational practices (see Freire, 1968, 1985, for a full discussion of the inhibitions present in education; also Giroux, 1992, 1994). While doctoral programs purport to be dealing with an interdisciplinary (or at least multi-disciplinary) subject, it is rare that interdisciplinary material is truly made available to students. The

common method of conveying alternative materials is to hire faculty
with degrees in various fields and assume that the teaching of "other
discipline" subjects imparts an interdisciplinary orientation to the
students. While we might quibble as to whether the result is multi-
disciplinary or interdisciplinary, the proof of the pudding would appear
to be its inclusion in the field. From that vantage point, I can find
integration of disciplinary materials in the fields of police and
correctional studies.[2] I cannot, however, say that for criminology.
Criminology appears to be as sociologically bound today as it was 30
years ago. That is not to say that materials from other disciplines are
not presented, indeed they are. However, they *way* they are presented is
rather suspect.[3] I realize there are exceptions to these generalities, and I
applaud those exceptions, but these comments reflect what *normally*
happens in graduate education in criminology.

Another educational problem is that our style of education itself
inhibits thinking abilities. For years, students are treated to an
educational scenario in which they get information from the teacher.
Among other things they learn that information comes *from* the teacher.
By the time they arrive at colleges and universities, most students have
learned it is inappropriate to think for themselves. Even at this new
level they continue to find this is true. Large class sizes and heavy
teaching loads in criminal justice and criminology departments are
normally sufficient to curb any impulse an instructor may have toward
encouraging students to think for themselves. Once these students are
in graduate school, they have learned that what instructors usually mean
by critical thinking is that they should think like the instructor, i.e., tell
the instructor what he or she told them. Indeed, it is my experience that
the most difficult thing in doctoral education is to actually convince
students that they, themselves, can think, discover, and be creative—
and that information doesn't have to come from the professor.

A final educational problem, particularly at the doctoral level, is
that students are forced into methodology and statistics courses that, on
the whole, overemphasize methodology and teach ideal types.
Unfortunately, this happens without a general understanding of the
philosophy of science and the place of method in epistemology that
might more properly provide a setting for quantitative techniques. As a
result, students definitively learn that error is bad and that systematic
objectivity is the hallmark of good work. What they do not learn well is
that *all* research has error and that *all* inquiry is partially subjective.
The true questions are what are the sources of error, how much error

can we tolerate, and in what ways are we subjectively asking questions and interpreting the data? The result of current education in methodology is that absolutely no one is more critical of information than a doctoral candidate.[4] Later in their scholarly careers they begin to learn the truth about error, but they rarely learn to think creatively. But the important piece of this education is that they learn that knowledge is tantamount to quantitative methodology—to create knowledge one must use empirical research tools. Unfortunately, the place of method in epistemic discussions is not a priority on the list of graduate school topics. And judging from the dominant work of the field, any creativity and self-initiated thoughts most criminological scholars might have once had have been successfully washed out by a flood of positivistic concern.[5]

Increasing Specialization

In addition to practices that directly discourage creativity, a century-old problem for virtually all disciplines has caught up with criminology and criminal justice: increasing specialization. It is no longer possible for one scholar to read published literature throughout the field. Indeed, a recent survey (Williams, McShane and Wagoner, 1996) found well over 120 journals in criminal justice alone, and the number of new books must exceed 200 every year. Several of my colleagues have expressed dismay at the quantity of materials, saying that they read very little of the broad journal literature, choosing instead to read in specialty areas

Overwhelming numbers of articles to be read is an obstacle to keeping track of the breadth of criminology and criminal justice, but it may not be the largest problem. The very focus on specialities is itself the culprit. In the past year, departments announced positions for criminal justice or criminological specialists who concentrate on corrections, police, courts, theory, law, sociology of law, minorities in the system, administration, security, and even methodology and statistics. While these announcements actually requested scholars who could teach in these areas, teaching interests usually reflect intellectual interests. Even students entering doctoral programs are advised to find a specialty.

Why is this a problem? I propose that a focus on specialities limits one's ability to think in larger terms. Perhaps a half century ago, criminology itself was an emerging specialty. At that point, there was a danger of forgetting that crime was merely one of the myriad forms of deviance (and of human behavior in general), all influenced by reaction to behavior. It would seem that this has come to pass, for many of today's scholars view crime as a unique entity. A recent plenary session with Robert Merton (1997) at the American Society of Criminology provides an instructive example. Reflecting on more than a half-century of his work, Merton viewed his role as a generalist who happened to do some work in criminology. Moreover, that work was really about deviance rather than crime *per se*. His contributions to the field clearly exemplify the value of a broader viewpoint.

Today's specialization problem transcends the earlier one. With scholars who specialize in small areas within the study of crime, one can now argue that even an appreciation of *crime* has been lost. How, for instance, does a specialist in methodology spend enough time reading and attempting to understand new theoretical concepts? This is, of course, a straw person question: we have had separate "researcher" and "theorists" categories for a long time. Neither is supposed to do well what the other does. Yet, we now have (for example) police management experts who not only do not appreciate what theorists do but even have lost an appreciation of the prosecutorial function, the system area closest to their specialty. Thus, the issue is no longer an ability to think creatively about behavior, a form of which is deviance (and a form of which is crime). The entire matter now becomes understanding and appreciation of a complex field. The definition of thinking in terms of the "big picture" has narrowed. And the narrower thinking becomes, the less likely one is to be creative.

Perhaps another way to put this problem is that we have begun to know more and more—but about less and less. Minute details are part of our specialization in minute areas. It is no small wonder that many of us do not really care about the work our colleagues do. This Balkanization of knowledge does seem to serve a status-seeking function, however, and one can gain a reputation within a small area. At the same time, the field pays the price in battles of theory versus theory and method versus method. Instead of status-competition, we might do better by choosing to view theory and method as imperfect, thereby providing a rationale for engaging in conversations with each other.

OVERCOMING THE PROBLEMS

I will elaborate more on the state of criminology in the next chapter. For now, however, I want to answer the logical critique which asks what can be done about these problems. While I am not sure that anyone has the answers, there are some general directions in which solutions might be found.

Encouraging an Appreciation of Qualitative Methodology

The first approach involves moving beyond the virtually exclusive dominance of quantitative methodology. It is the dominance with which I am concerned not the methodology *per se*. The social sciences simply need to spend more time closer to their subjects, and we need to learn from those subjects. Informative directions for qualitative research are to begin to know and to understand the feelings and thoughts of humans. That is, we need to know how humans process information, integrate it with their experiences, and use the result to create behavior. Jeff Ferrell (1997) refers to this as "criminological verstehen." He expounds an understanding of criminality that is necessarily grounded in "the situated logic and emotion of crime" (1997:109). Such approaches require criminologists to almost *be there* when crimes are committed or, if not actually there, as close as possible in time and space.

By this logic, surveys and secondary data will not do. Simply looking at external influences and behavior will not allow an understanding of how and why things occur, but it does allow some degree of aggregate prediction. And that is precisely why we have misunderstood humans. Until such time as we find ways of accurately quantifying feelings and thought processes, researchers need to expand on the ability to locate those feelings and thoughts. All of this, of course, means that we need to encourage qualitative research capable of producing results that can ultimately be incorporated into quantitative methodology. For now, we need more of the qualitative sort.

Interdisciplinary Education

Because we have a tendency to focus on the concepts of a single discipline, criminology and criminal justice must begin to foster true interdisciplinary education.[6] This means that students and future colleagues should develop an appreciation of the value of knowledge from various disciplines and feel comfortable with incorporating that knowledge into their work. This, however, is not an easy task, mostly because it demands that current reductionist thinking be set aside in order to begin the process. If people could do so easily, then the problem would not now exist. Perhaps the best we can do for a while is to prepare students with multi-disciplinary graduate work and hope that they integrate the materials themselves. Even to do this, instructors must attempt to set aside their biases toward other disciplines. Otherwise, the communicated materials will approximate what we are doing now.

Non-Linear Thinking

Just as we need interdisciplinary thinking, we also need non-linear thinking (and analysis). Researchers and theorists need to be encouraged to understand causality in new ways and approach problems with new tools.[7] In short, we can no longer afford to assume the social world is neatly laid out for us in an end-to-end manner. One piece of causality that probably affects much of what we do is the commonly-accepted part of the Millsian schema that a presumed cause must precede a presumed effect. This is often interpreted as temporal *and proximate* precedence. While John Stuart Mills clearly did not express the causal condition as temporal proximity, the implication is that a real cause should come before the effect but probably not too far before it. After all, where in time does one stop in searching for a preceding variable to be inferred as a cause? The implication is that causes should be temporally *near* (temporal proximity) their presumed effect (causal problems will be covered in more detail in Chapter Three).

Thus, a second problem emerges. There is the tendency to mistake temporal proximity to an effect as its cause. Some philosophers of causality have even argued that humans are conditioned through evolution to view temporally proximate variables as causes (Michotte, 1963). While it is true that modern science has expanded the causal universe with probabilistic approaches, it is also likely that the variables we choose to measure for our research in this probabilistic universe tend to be those with proximate qualities. Researchers need to begin to think in terms of multi-disciplinary variables that interact in various non-linear formulations.

Appreciating Subjectivity

Subjectivity is another misunderstood concept in research. The hallowed goal is pure objectivity; thus any subjectivity is viewed as bad among quantitative researchers. At the same time, virtually all methods texts contain a chapter on the place of values and ethics in research. One of the most widely used texts (Babbie, 1995) even has an extensive discussion on the inevitability of values entering into various research stages. With this in mind, it makes sense to view subjectivity as *part* of research, to appreciate subjectivity and *use* it to advantage. One way to do this is to follow the objective model and incorporate subjectivity as error—but error that is estimated and understood rather than mentioned and then ignored. Objective models of social reality have not been able to generate accurate (nor even necessarily, reliable) predictions of social action or behavior. One reason is that what is unknown (a major component of the "error term") may affect what is known in multiple ways. The non-objective components of reality (a source of the "unknown" in objective models) deserve inclusion if for no other reason than to acknowledge their existence. We have been able to produce methods of estimating and examining latent structures; surely we can incorporate subjectivity into that latency.

A second method of incorporating subjectivity is to understand that the subjects of our research have their own subjectivity and that subjectivity, far from being something that obscures "real" variables, governs the way in which living takes place. Put another way, subjectivity is the reality by which people act (a lesson from symbolic interactionism), including both research subjects and the researchers who study them. A form of subjectivity that combines both researcher and researched is probably necessary in order for social scientists to understand social reality (see, for instance, Richard Quinney's recent work [1988, 1991, 1993, 1995] relating Zen to criminology). If we fail to appreciate this, then we fail to understand human existence.

Expansive Thinking

The final issue in this section is that of limited thinking. On the one hand, limited thinking may be in part derived from specialization, either in subject matter or in methodology. On the other hand, there is ample evidence that such thinking is not restricted to the issue of specialization. Indeed, it appears that most people tend to be more limited than expansive thinkers. Graduate students, however, should be capable of dealing with wider issues and seeing information in wider context. To make sure this happens, educational programs need to infuse material on creative thinking into course work. While I realize that existing curricula are such that there is scarcely room for new materials, most graduate programs are continually in a state of "revision." Some treatment of creativity would seem justified. After all, that *is* one of the things that supposedly moves science along.

We also need to move beyond simplistic conceptions that theories compete with each other. The fact is that most theories are not explaining the same things. Thus, students need to be taught to look for similarities *and* differences between theories, to integrate materials from various approaches and to use those materials in ways that seem reasonable (rather than only the way that the original theorist used them).

Lastly, the propensity to use dichotomies should be discouraged, mostly because dualistic frameworks rarely describe reality and encourage thinking in terms of opposites. As was noted earlier, our thinking tends to set up theories in a form of competition. A framework based on dichotomies encourages and furthers this approach. By viewing reality as infinitely more complex, we may come to see our explanations as pieces of the same puzzle.

A MORE CREATIVE PERSPECTIVE

It is well and good to express these concerns and even suggest some limited solutions. But what specifically would assist creativity in criminology and criminal justice? First, I would make the observation that organization itself limits creativity. We create structured approaches to the world specifically to enhance our understanding of it. Yet I am not sure that we *understand* more—although I do believe that we are busy *explaining* more. Whether that explanation is conducive to understanding crime and criminals is another matter entirely. The more structured criminology and criminal justice become, the more likely it is that we will severely limit our thinking. As a result, it may well behoove us to be less structured and organized, at least occasionally. Lacking that, we may find ways to organize differently.

A New Exemplar

One notion of organization in the sciences is contained in the concept of a paradigm, a term most closely associated with Thomas Kuhn. In

The Structure of Scientific Revolutions Kuhn used the word "paradigm" many different ways and, as it turns out, social scientists seized not on his concept of paradigms but on his discussion of what Masterman was later to term "metaparadigms" (Masterman, 1970)—disciplinary approaches to problems. Years after that publication, Kuhn (1977) clarified what he meant by *paradigm*—a puzzle-solving and analytical exemplar demonstrating how to perceive and approach a problem. To demonstrate the use of paradigms, he used the example of problems in the back of each chapter of a physics text (the rolling of a ball down an inclined plane to demonstrate friction). Following that lead and clarifying what I intend in this book, I would like to specify an exemplar for this work in terms of our basic disciplinary questions.

Current work largely focuses on the deviant or criminal act or crime rates as a measure of criminal acts. Even those who study victimization are still tied to an objective criminal act. In a recent critique and research study, Terance Miethe and David McDowall (1993) noted this problem and incorporated the effect of context on criminal victimization in an attempt to move away from a straightforward emphasis on acts. In short, the main focus of contemporary mainstream criminology is embodied in the chase to explain the criminal act and criminal behavior from an *objective* perspective that is outside of the framework of those who *experience* that act. The common exemplar is to demonstrate research into crime by employing quantitative methods that collect data to be translated into numbers suitable for statistical analysis. These exemplars are found in such various places as textbooks that evaluate theory based on empirical evidence, virtually any published article on crime and criminals, and introductory criminology and criminal justice textbooks that present crime and criminality as a series of variables.

I propose that we refocus the exemplar so that other forms of investigation become acceptable (Bruce Arrigo [1995] has similarly proposed changing the stock question of criminology; see his article for an elaborated discussion). Such a change is subtle but necessary to get on with an understanding of the criminal event and its effect on people. Two things are necessary in this refocusing: we must get beyond the purely quantitative, "objective" approaches to evidence and we must appreciate the non-linearity of the criminal experience. In short, I would prefer to ask *"What is the deviant or criminal experience?,"* rather than ask questions about the criminal act. Perhaps some would even view this as a question about "what *constructs* the deviant or criminal experience?"

Implications of a Change in the Exemplar

This simple change re-orients two basic perceptual directions: what information to collect and how to interpret that information. First, it tells us to collect information about the *experience*. This requires information from the *viewpoint of the individual* as well as from the *viewpoint of the victim* and of *reactors*. Jock Young (1992) has elaborated on these components of crime using a concept that he calls the "square of crime." He identifies "four definitional elements of crime: a victim, an offender, formal control and informal control" (Young, 1992:27). The elements operate in time and space to create an environment for crime. A primary advantage of the square of crime is that it redirects traditional attention paid to the offender and places crime in a multifaceted network with multiple operating factors. Young's conception provides a larger list of *questions* about crime than is common with most criminological theories. It appears that this expanded view integrates social reaction, structural conditions and offender motivation, thus expanding criminological awareness of the various factors at play in a criminal event. But critical criminologists are not the only ones who have recognized the need to expand the awareness of crime. For instance, Terance Miethe and Robert Meier (1995) have also recently bemoaned the focus on a criminal act. They present a theoretical position based on victim and offender interaction which leads to a particular social context and thus to crime.

The second reorientation suggests that *both* objective and subjective interpretations have value for understanding. Tangential issues from asking "what is the experience?" include establishing how the experience affects other people (reactors) and what relationships exist with the physical environment. Finally, the change should facilitate explanations that contribute to understanding crime.

Both basic perceptual directions change the traditional approach to perceiving deviance. First, our common exemplars are bound to positivistic empiricism: we need *objective* data in order to understand the world. The existing approach attempts to explain the deviant *act*, which is an objective phenomenon. Therefore, although there is traditionally no inherent prohibition to requesting subjective motivational information from the subject, data are more likely to be collected around that act and the objective motivations of the subject.[8] Second, the individual is currently denigrated in favor of *groups* and aggregate data. While such an approach is both proper and disciplinarily correct for sociologists (see Jensen, 1981:7), it simply doesn't make much sense to study criminals and criminal acts from only one perspective. This brings to mind Cooley's old example of contrasting General Grant's view of his army from the top of a hill with the view obtained by looking each person in the face. He argued that the phenomenon was the same, but the information obtained was different. I am arguing that without doing *both*, viewing the individual soldiers and having an overall view of the army in which they exist, there is no possible understanding of the phenomenon.

Does this mean that we must achieve both levels of viewing a phenomenon at the same time? My answer is "yes and no." If we want to understand both criminals and crime, it is necessary to develop information on both subjective and objective realities and both individual and structural factors. This may be done separately—using the existing skills of researchers—and then conceptually reconstructing evidence into a more holistic picture of reality. Such an approach is not entirely satisfactory because it involves the combining of two different "pictures," thereby requiring assumptions about the proper way the final picture should fit together. The preferred approach would be to construct a research design that takes advantage of *all* the information at once (both qualitative and quantitative at the same time). In this way, reality emerges as a whole rather than in a reconstructed, piecemeal fashion. Unfortunately, this approach requires a great degree of skill in two different techniques and not many researchers have such skill. At the least this argues for required courses in qualitative methods at the graduate level and a tacit recognition from the graduate faculty of the value of those techniques.

OVERVIEW OF THE BOOK

As should be now evident, the text to follow includes both a critique of contemporary positivist-based criminology and an alternative to that perspective. Rather than offering a "new" theory, I have chosen to offer a new orienting perspective, a different way of perceiving reality, under which existing theories may be used and reinterpreted. Before approaching that perspective, however, the next three chapters review theoretical concerns and focus on the critique.

Chapter Two provides an overview of criminological theorizing from the 1970s to the present. The most popular theories and those with interesting insights (not necessarily the same theories) are briefly examined and critiqued from the perspective of their ability to provide clues into and/or appreciate the complexity of criminological reality.

Chapter Three continues much of what has been begun in this introductory chapter. In it, I present an overview of the theoretical field, particularly the work of the past two decades, and review the similarities and differences between the various perspectives. Following that, an attempt is made to determine why various theories are popular at different times, dwelling at length on issues presented by the concept of competing theories, fashions and fads and paradigms. The final section examines reasons for the failure of theory to adequately deal with the reality of crime.

The fourth chapter examines the use of concepts and the way we way we formulate and measure them. It begins with a discussion of the way in which definitions of crime have hampered work, continues with an examination of how critical explanatory variables have been conceived and measured, and concludes with some suggestions for improving measurement.

Chapter Five deals with methodology and subjectivity. It first looks at methodologies of contemporary criminology and then examines the uses of subjectivity in criminology. The initial discussion deals with our overemphasis on empirical, quantitative methods. Following that there is a review of the degree of substance in our data, the orientation toward aggregate information and survey methodology and the concept of error. The second major section focuses on the presence of values in method and theory, noting that subjectivity exists within objective methods. A case is then made for introducing subjectivity into criminological method and distinguishes between the perspectives of the actor and those of the researcher. The chapter concludes with a brief discussion of the effect of language on values and interpretation.

Beginning with the theoretical perspective of the book, Chapter Six discusses the need for theoretical models that are capable of dealing with complexity. The major forms of complexity theory in the natural sciences today are based on chaos theory. The general history and concepts of chaos theory are explored, with attention paid to the emergence of patterns and shapes from seemingly random data. A specific form of chaos theory, self-organized criticality, is discussed.

The final section further examines self-organized criticality theory and explains its main concepts.

Chapter Seven introduces the metatheoretical perspective that will be drawn from the chaos theory concepts. After specifying what portions of the original chaos-based version of self-organized criticality theory are adaptable, the new perspective on criminal behavior (critical-incident metatheory) is generally advanced and its major concepts explained. Ending the chapter, the way in which the theory deals with social reaction is discussed and behavior and reaction are combined.

Chapter Eight continues the discussion of the metatheory, adding to the previous general discussion with specifics needed to understand its complexity. Various individual points are discussed and examples are provided, along with some exploration of how the metatheoretical specifics reflect on reality.

Chapter Nine deals with the implications of critical-incident metatheory for existing method and unit theories. It begins with the reason for presenting a metatheory rather than a unit theory and makes general suggestions for re-orienting criminology. Then the chapter discusses a range of specific issues, including prediction, how current theories might fit into the new concepts, levels of explanation and integration of theories. The final section examines the use of subjectivity under the metatheory.

The final chapter offers a rationale on the purpose of the commentary and metatheory and answers some anticipated criticisms. In addition, it offers some concluding comments about instilling the use of imagination so that creativity will become more common among criminological scholars.

NOTES

1. While I do not intend to extend these arguments to the social sciences in general, it is most likely that the same can be said of virtually all of the social science disciplines.

2. Actually, a case can be made for inclusion of criminal justice system studies in the criminological framework. One of the primary messages of the societal reaction approach was that one had to understand the agency reaction to crime as one aspect of criminality.

3. In most cases, biological and psychological explanations of criminality are presented in a highly critical fashion and labeled reductionistic. Sociological perspectives are also critiqued, but not quite as critically and

usually with a bias toward some favorite theory of the moment. The message is clear: sociological theories are better, if for no other reason than the fact that they deal with social aggregates and thereby predict *rates* of behavior. In fairness, though this is the way some view the proper role of sociology (e.g., Babbie, 1995:30), there are other sociologies such as those embodied in the symbolic interactionist perspective that do *not* focus on social structures and rates of behavior. Pitirim Sorokin's classic pronouncement was that "Sociology is interested only in those aspects of social phenomena and their relations which are repeated either in time or in space or both; which consequently exhibit some uniformity of constancy or typicality" (1928:760). Other statements by Lester Ward (1899) and George Lundberg (1964) suggest that, prior to the past two decades, it was common to view sociology as a general social science. It seems that many of today's criminologists have taken these sorts of statements to mean that sociological phenomena are properly *statistical* social phenomena.

4. Jeff Walker brought to my attention that this group would potentially vie with another—manuscript reviewers—for the honor.

5. It is also true that the gate-keeping function served by orientation of major journals serves to continually emphasize the "correct" form of knowledge.

6. This is by no means a new issue. Marvin Wolfgang has long advocated a separate disciplinary identity for criminology (see Wolfgang, 1963), yet he acknowledges the importance of sociology. Ray Jeffery has campaigned for the acceptance of other disciplines in criminology (1978). Arnie Binder (1987), in an article examining the interdisciplinarity of criminology, favored the interdisciplinary approach yet made a good case that forays by non-sociological disciplines have remained unidisciplinary. On the other side, Ron Akers, in his 1992 presidential address before the Southern Sociological Society, argued forcefully that criminology belonged in sociology, and sociology was, and should be, the center of criminology (Akers, 1992). However, Akers views both individuals and social structure as the proper focus of sociology (1981:177-178) and acknowledges that other disciplines have become part of criminology. Similarly, Charles Wellford (1991) appears to believe that criminology is a sociological enterprise, but, at the same time, he wants an organizational separation between the two.

7. For a comprehensive treatment of the issues behind causality in the social sciences, I refer readers to Bruce DiCristina's *Method in Criminology: A Philosophical Primer* (New York, NY: Harrow and Heston, 1995). The book has an excellent discussion of causation in general, probability, and falsification.

8. Of late, there is a tendency to ignore motivational information entirely in favor of a fully objective approach to the act. Indeed, some contemporary approaches which favor explaining criminal acts from the perspective of the victim either dismiss the criminal motivation altogether or arbitrarily ascribe criminal motivation to a rational choice.

REFERENCES

Akers, Ronald L. (1992). Linking sociology and its specialities: The case of criminology. *Social Forces* 71: 1–16.

Akers, Ronald L. (1981). Reflections of a social behaviorist on behavioral sociology. *The American Sociologist* 16: 177–180.

Arrigo, Bruce A. (1995). The peripheral core of law and criminology: On postmodern social theory and conceptual integration. *Justice Quarterly* 12: 447–472.

Babbie, Earl (1995). *The Practice of Social Research*, 7th ed. Belmont, CA: Wadsworth.

Binder, Arnold (1987). Criminology: Discipline or an interdiscipline? *Issues in Integrative Studies* 5: 41–67.

DiCristina, Bruce (1995). *Method in Criminology: A Philosophical Primer.* New York, NY: Harrow and Heston.

Ferrell, Jeff (1997). Criminological *verstehen*: Inside the immediacy of crime. *Justice Quarterly* 14: 3–23.

Freire, Paulo (1968). *Pedagogy of the Oppressed.* New York, NY: Seabury.

Freire, Paulo (1985). *The Politics of Education.* South Hadley, MA: Bergin and Garvey.

Gibbons, Don C. (1994). *Talking about Crime and Criminals: Problems and Issues in Theory Development in Criminology.* Englewood Cliffs, NJ: Prentice Hall.

Giroux, Henry A. (1992). *Border Crossings.* New York, NY: Routledge.

Giroux, Henry A. (1994). *Between Borders: Pedagogy and the Politics of Cultural Studies.* New York, NY: Routledge.

Gouldner, Alvin W. (1970). *The Coming Crisis of Western Sociology.* New York, NY: Basic Books.

Jeffery, C. Ray (1978). Criminology as an interdisciplinary behavioral science. *Criminology* 16: 149–169.

Jensen, Gary F. (1981). The sociology of delinquency: Current issues. Pp. 7–19 in Gary F. Jensen (ed.) *Sociology of Delinquency: Current Issues.* Beverly Hills, CA: Sage.

Kuhn, Thomas S. (1964, 1970). *The Structure of Scientific Revolutions*. Chicago, IL: University of Chicago Press.

Kuhn, Thomas S. (1977). Second thoughts on paradigms. Pp. 293–319 in Thomas S. Kuhn (ed.) *The Essential Tension*. Chicago, IL: University of Chicago Press.

Lundberg, George A. (1964). *Foundations of Sociology*. New York, NY: McKay.

Masterman, Margaret (1970). The nature of a paradigm. Pp. 59–90 in Imre Lakatos and Alan Musgrave (eds.), *Criticism and the Growth of Knowledge*. Cambridge, UK: Cambridge University Press.

Merton, Robert K. (1997). On the evolving synthesis of differential association and anomie theory: A perspective from the sociology of science. *Criminology* 35: 517-525.

Michotte, Alan (1963). *The Perception of Causality*. New York, NY: Basic Books.

Miethe, Terance D., and David McDowall (1993). Contextual effects in models of criminal victimization. *Social Forces* 71: 741–760.

Miethe, Terance D., and Robert F. Meier (1995). *Crime and Its Social Context: Toward an Integrated Theory of Offenders, Victims, and Situations*. Albany, NY: State University of New York Press.

Mills, C. Wright (1959). *The Sociological Imagination*. New York, NY: Oxford University Press.

Quinney, Richard (1988). Beyond the interpretative: The way of awareness. *Sociological Inquiry* 58: 101–116.

Quinney, Richard (1991). The way of peace: On crime, suffering and service. In Harold E. Pepinsky and Richard Quinney (eds.) *Criminology as Peacemaking*. Bloomington, IN: Indiana University Press.

Quinney, Richard (1993). A life of crime: Criminology and public policy as peacemaking. *Journal of Crime and Justice* 16: 3–9.

Quinney, Richard (1995). Socialist humanism and the problem of crime. *Crime, Law and Social Change* 23: 147–156.

Sorokin, Pitirim (1928). *Contemporary Sociological Theories*. New York, NY: Harper.

Ward, Lester A. (1899). *Outlines of Sociology*. New York: Macmillan.

Wellford, Charles F. (1991). Graduate programs in criminology and criminal justice: What are our needs? *The Criminologist* 16: 4–5.

Wellford, Charles F. (1989). Towards an integrated theory of criminal behavior. Pp. 119–128 in Steven F. Messner, Marvin D. Krohn and Allen E. Liska (eds.) *Theoretical Integration in the Study of Deviance and Crime:*

Problems and Prospects. Albany, NY: State University of New York Press.

Williams, Frank P., III, Marilyn D. McShane, and Carl P. Wagoner (1996). The ratings of criminal justice journals: A survey of ACJS members. *American Journal of Criminal Justice* 19: 301–324.

Wolfgang, Marvin E. (1963). Criminology and the criminologist. *Journal of Criminal Law, Criminology, and Police Science* 54: 155–162.

Young, Jock (1992). Ten points of realism. Pp. 24–68 in Jock Young and Roger Matthews (eds.) *Rethinking Criminology: The Realist Debate.* London: Sage.

CHAPTER TWO

Recent Criminological Theorizing

This chapter reviews, evaluates and reflects on the enterprise of contemporary criminological theory from 1970 to the present. The intention is to locate the flow of ideas over time and determine what has been added to our understanding of crime and criminals. In doing this, it makes sense to focus on the theories that have been (or are) the most popular, because those theories reflect (or create) the dominant view of the field. For this reason I am not concerned with a comprehensive review or even representative coverage, although there will be occasional discussion of less popular theories that have made interesting and/or divergent contributions.[1] The key question to be answered is whether various contributions to criminological knowledge have led us any closer to an appreciation of a complex reality.

THE THEORIES OF THE 1970s

Labeling and Conflict Theories

The decade of the 1970s began as a liberal period and ended with a transition into conservatism. The carry-over of 1960s liberalism (and even radicalism) made labeling and conflict theories popular, particularly with graduate students. There was much to examine in politically sensitive crime theory. The U.S. government was heavy handed in dealing with civil unrest and Viet Nam war protests. Media frequently relayed stories of governmental malfeasance and misfeasance. For most criminologists, it was clear that crime was defined and constructed politically—the problem was determining exactly what this meant. Those criminologists who were more critical were convinced that the political construction of crime was *the* key ingredient to the crime recipe. Foremost among these were Richard Quinney, who contributed several major works during the period (c.f., *The Social Reality of Crime*; *Critique of Legal Order*; *Class, Status, and Crime*) and Ian Taylor, Paul Walton, and Jock Young, who provided critical criminologists with a resounding critique of mainstream criminology (*The New Criminology*). While there were many contributors to critical criminology (and a substantial number of scholars are still contributing), most graduate students shook off their enthusiasm for the romantic notions of radicalism once they got their degrees and retreated to more traditional versions of criminology.

More conservative criminologists saw the political construction of crime as merely a legislative enactment of public desires. Although they seemed to recognize the contribution of special interest groups to that legislation, the vast bulk of criminal law was aligned with public conceptions of harm. Therefore, definitions of "crime" still matched harmful and socially undesirable behavior (the issue of defining crime is treated in Chapter Four). If drawn at all to 1960s liberalism, these criminologists adopted pluralist versions of conflict (though not for long).

What did the liberal 1970s contribute to complexity? Clearly, the major contribution was an insistence that criminal behavior be placed in context. The "older" labeling concept of hidden criminality yielded to a more complex version of social reaction where the political definition of crime determined who would be reacted to, the form of reaction and the historical context of crime. In short, critical criminologists contributed a "non-criminal" side of the crime event. The more radical ones also repainted the criminal as the capitalist, financier, or politician who made or influenced laws on their own behalf, to the detriment of the working person. Such contributions enriched the overall picture of crime. Yet they were uniformly applied from a one-dimensional perspective, and the actor was ignored (unless the crime was political or white collar). The problem of harm from street crime was glossed over. Nevertheless, the "other" side of the crime picture was a powerful message. C. Ray Jeffery (1971:256–257) captured the essence of the total crime picture with his comment that an explanation of crime required a theory of crime (political theory), a theory of behavior and, finally, a theory of criminal behavior. The degree to which this seemingly obvious message had an effect on criminology is debatable, however. Conservative criminology remained in the mainstream, and most of the discussion returned to a vision of the criminal.

Social Control and Social Learning Theories

In case the discussion above seems to suggest that *only* critical movements were taking place in the 1970s, it is worthwhile to remember that there were subtle changes afoot of a different nature. Religion became more important for many and the "born-again" movement grew throughout the decade. The cynicism about government fostered by the Vietnam War and protest movements was further advanced by Watergate. A mid-1970s gasoline crisis heightened economic concerns. These events and others contributed to a growing mood of conservatism and, linked with a public concerned with crime rates that had been growing throughout the period, made it easy to return to the study of criminals. Two theories, both derived from the late 1960s, facilitated this movement.

Social control theory as advanced by Travis Hirschi (1969) was to become the most popular criminological perspective by mid-decade. Spurred on by disenchantment with the Chicago School and anomie theories, criminologists were looking for an alternative to perspectives that blamed society for criminal behavior without really giving up a social perspective. In this search, they found an appealing substitute in the social control notion of an individual who is somehow cut loose from the bonds and controls of society, thus free to commit crime. It was possible to leave society in the picture, yet focus on the individual and, in particular, the contribution of parents. Hirschi's four posited elements of the bond—attachment, commitment, involvement and belief— provided a way for researchers to examine the "glue" of societal order and conformity. The question before criminologists was how to strengthen the bonds of an individual so that criminal urges could be fought off. In fact, there was no need even to explain criminal urges or pushes toward criminality. In social control theory, people are naturally self-interested and potentially unrestrained. It is the restraints on their behavior that need to be explained. In other words, crime is "natural," conformity is unnatural. In such a world, the causes of crime devolve to improper socialization of various types.

Social learning theory (Burgess and Akers, 1966; Akers, 1973) was another popular criminological perspective of the period. The blend of differential association with psychologically-based operant and social learning theories gave new life to Chicago School concepts. The core of the theory was that previously learned behavior (derived from individual experiences and cultural definitions) affected future behavior. Consequently, the theory is perhaps the most testable perspective in criminology. Why it did not eclipse social control theory is a matter of speculation. One reason might be its identification with psychology, while criminology is largely a sociological discipline. Another might be that it extended Sutherland's theory of differential association during a period in which the older theories were in decline. For whatever reason, social learning theory remained a well-cited but secondary theory throughout the decade. Its contributions included a reminder that criminal behavior was a product of complex experiences and situations. The chief architect of social learning, Ron Akers, was able to couch the situational aspects (shared experiences and cultural definitions) in a subcultural milieu, but the theory remained at heart an individually-focused explanation of the process of becoming deviant.

What did these two theories contribute to understanding the complexity of criminal event? First, it should be noted that because both theories were derived from earlier perspectives, their contributions might be seen as limited. Yet, both had something new to say. Social control theory reminded us that there is a connection between conformity and deviance, thus suggesting that deviance was not a unique form of behavior. But in the end, social control reaffirmed the importance of social institutions and its complexity lesson was largely lost. Social learning theory, on the other hand, echoed the lack of uniqueness in criminal behavior *and* told us that both the cultural milieu and personal experiences were important to predicting behavior. Its emphasis on individual differences in learning had potential for leading criminologists in new directions.

Feminist Theories

Feminist theory, derived from the writings of the late 1960s, developed throughout the 1970s. Most of the work in criminology was a continuation of ideas present in radical thought. However, there were two major alternatives to explaining female crime that took a nonradical course. In *Sisters in Crime* (1975) Freda Adler argued that changes in female criminality were the product of changes in the social roles of women. Based on observations about the women's liberation movement, Adler's theory posited that American society had grown progressively more receptive to females in the workforce, thereby giving females greater freedom. As women assume more assertive positions in society and adopt more traditionally "male" roles and statuses, their behavior will reflect more masculine characteristics. Women will therefore commit more traditionally male crimes, such as violent crimes and white-collar crimes, and the overall rate of female crime will increase. As the gender gap narrows, the behavior of women and men, both legitimate and illegitimate, will be more alike.

The second perspective was presented by Rita James Simon (1976). This was a variation on the women's liberation approach that focused on opportunities available to females. Simon argued that the form of female criminality is a product of social, familial and occupational structures in the lives of women. Consequently, changes in the traditional roles of women were also a key to the hypothesis that, over time, women will be involved in more employment-related crimes. However, instead of focusing on changes in the personal roles of women in society or on the consideration of behaviors as either feminine or masculine, her perspective simply looks at the opportunities women have available to participate in crime. In the past, Simon argues, limited participation in the labor force blocked women's access to opportunities to commit crimes such as fraud, embezzlement and grand larceny. For example, as clerks and tellers, women in business and banking were too closely supervised to steal successfully. However, as women move into the ranks of executives, managers and accountants, there is greater access to more covert theft opportunities.

These theories, while rather simplistic in their approach to criminality, contributed to a rising consciousness soon to flourish as gender studies. They also added to the criminological mix, in that mainstream theories tended to assume that female criminality was either not worth explaining or that females were merely part of explanations of male criminality. As to the question of added complexity, feminist theories in general tended to reflect critical/radical thought or, in the case of the Adler/Simon perspectives, were no more understanding of complex social reality than their male theory counterparts.

Victim-Based Rational Theories

The continued trend toward conservatism in the late 1970s yielded a growing concern with crime as having gotten out of control. The essence of the period, for criminal justice and crime, was a time of crime control and punitive policies. Criminals were seen as people who were bad (Wilson, 1975) or who purposefully decided to commit criminal acts. They were to be punished because they "deserved it." Victims' rights were introduced into the criminal justice system, and victims were asked for their opinion about sentences. The new victim surveys provided new information on a side of the crime equation that had been largely forgotten: the victim.

In this climate, two new theoretical articles appeared. Both were focused on victim data and both attempted to explain crime by reference to lifestyles and routine activities (Hindelang, Gottfredson, and Garofalo, 1978; Cohen and Felson, 1979).[2] Interestingly, both perspectives assumed that criminals were rational creatures. The idea was to describe the factors that one would expect to find in aggregate decisions to commit crime.

Routine Activities Theory

Larry Cohen and Marcus Felson's (1979) routine activities perspective was initially viewed as a very practical look at crime. However, it gained in popularity and became a major perspective of the 1980s. They combined interests in the new victimology with a new ecological crime-prevention approach. As already noted, they assumed that decisions involved in victimization events were rational.

Routine activities theory argues that the volume of criminal offenses is related to the nature of everyday patterns of social interaction. As the pattern of social interaction changes, so does the number of crimes. Cohen and Felson emphasized the nature of routine activities (common social activities) as an essential part of everyday life. As social change disrupts or changes routine activities, social disorganization can occur and crime opportunities may increase. The victimization event has three major areas of focus: a motivated offender, a suitable target, and an absence of a capable guardian. If one of these components is missing, crime is not likely to happen. Because of routine activities, suitable victims (or targets) are found more frequently in some settings than others.

Lifestyle Theory

Michael Hindelang, Michael Gottfredson, and James Garofalo (1978) wanted to know why certain groups of people were at greater risk of being victims of crime than others. Their answer was that patterned activities, or lifestyles, of individuals led to differential victimization rates. These lifestyles were characterized by daily functions involving both work and leisure activities.

Lifestyles are influenced by three basic elements: social roles played by people in society, position in the social structure, and rational decisions about which behaviors are desirable. Based on one's social role and structural position, decisions can be made to restrict routine behaviors to relatively safe ones or to accept risk. Risks can be decreased or increased beyond the levels normally expected for one's group by the conscious decisions individuals make to engage in certain lifestyles.

Contribution to Complexity

How did routine activities and lifestyle theories affect understandings of complexity? Clearly, they promised to add a dimension, the victim, to what had previously been a discussion focused on the criminal (of course, labeling and conflict had already added the reactor dimension). From this perspective, these theories had great potential, suggesting that a criminal event was a combination of factors affecting the criminal, the environmental situation at the moment of criminal opportunity, and the decisions made by potential victims. The subsequent focus on criminals as rational decision-makers, however, diminished the chances of all three elements being incorporated into a complex whole.

This gaining and losing of information was not solely a problem for rational theories. Unfortunately, the mainstream sociological focus on social events and factors seemed to serve as blinders for most criminologists of the 1970s. This, and the emergence of the two dominant theories (social control and social learning) during the 1960s, is central to what some critics have referred to as a dearth of theory during the 1970s and early 1980s (Williams, 1984; Meier, 1985; Whitehead, 1986; Braithwaite, 1989a; Walters, 1989). The lone exception seemed to be the theorizing present in radical and critical theories (Chambliss, 1975; Gordon, 1973; Quinney, 1977; Spitzer, 1975; Tifft, 1979), where there was a progressive trend that incorporated previously developed materials.[3] At the most fundamental level, however, criminology exhibited little new understanding of criminal reality. The potential for incorporating complexity was largely ignored by mainstream criminologists during the period.

THEORIZING IN THE 1980s and 1990s[4]

All in all, the 1980s represented a period of time when U.S. society was punitively oriented and relatively intolerant. Several political and power groups emerged, each advocating their own position with little concern for others. Each group told us why others were not to be trusted, were doing bad things to us, or had incorrect values. Against this backdrop, scholars were gaining ideas and reacting to popular positions.

The lack of new theoretical ideas continued from the 1970s until the mid-1980s. Toward the end of the decade, however, a concern with theoretical criminology seemed to grow. That concern was balanced with popular, anti-theoretical positions taken by some writers on crime (beginning with James Q. Wilson in 1975) and administrators in government criminal justice circles. Just as rehabilitation was pronounced "dead" in the 1970s, so was criminological theorizing pronounced a waste of money and effort in the 1980s. It would suffice, we were told, that evil people would be held responsible for their actions and punished. Our needs were simple: More efficient criminal justice systems, more prisons, and more police on the street.

If people were indeed evil or self-centered the problem was not how to explain the background factors of criminality but instead to explain how criminals thought differently. The criminal personality theory of Yochelson and Samenow (1976) began the cognitive movement, but most criminologists were still sociologically oriented enough to want a perspective grounded in social phenomena.

Finally, just as self-report studies had created a new form of evidence for crime theories, the emergence of national victimization studies in 1972 provided yet another set of facts to be explained. Victimization statistics, by 1980, had become the new, intriguing information about crime and, by the end of the decade, would be the mainstay of criminological evidence. And, as was probably inevitable, these statistics provided the fuel for the new rationalist theories and a new paradigm for criminology.

Rationalist Theories

Rational Choice

Rationalist theories seem to share a common belief that criminal rationality is hedonistic and that certain background factors lead to that result. This alone, however, cannot uniquely account for crime since the perspective would hold that most of life's decisions are made on the basis of hedonistic principles (at least they are if one believes the explanations of behavioristic psychology). The primary element introduced by rational choice theorists, such as Derek Cornish and Ronald Clarke (1986), is that the decision to commit a crime is a product of expected effort, anticipated rewards, and assumed costs. If effort and costs are high, while rewards are relatively low, there will be no crime. Derived from economics, this is the same as saying that humans wish to maximize profit and minimize loss. It is also a virtual repetition of the utilitarian philosophy of Jeremy Bentham; therefore, nothing particularly new is added by this perspective. While the concept of behavior as a product of a rational calculation of risk and rewards has an intuitive appeal, in practice there is little evidence that humans make decisions in that fashion (Paternoster *et al.*, 1983; Tunnell, 1992). Nonetheless, rational choice theories were relatively popular among criminologists and those in governmental circles during the 1980s. Their focus on the offender and emphasis on "willful" decision-making do not contribute to an understanding of a complex reality and, in fact, offer a more simplified reality than most alternative theories.

Another form of rational choice theory is deterrence, an old classical-era perspective that made a comeback during the period. Modifications of the basic legal version of deterrence combined informal social variables into a generic version of "cost calculation" (see Grasmick and Green, 1980; Meier and Johnson, 1977; Williams, 1985; Green, 1989; Williams and Hawkins, 1989; Grasmick and Bursik, 1990; Nagin and Paternoster, 1991). These versions present the essence of the legal reward/punishment and add the effect of social sanctions. While more complex than the traditional deterrence model, they still focus on the offender's rational decision-making capacity and simply add informal, social variables into the calculation mix.

Cognitive Rationalism

A second cognitive perspective has been offered by Glen Walters and Thomas White (1989a) and elaborated in a 1990 book by Walters. They argue that criminal behavior is the product of faulty, irrational thinking and deny that environmental factors determine criminal behavior (although they do note that environment serves to limit options). Focusing on "lifestyle" or career criminals, Walters and White point out that these individuals are characterized in most, if not all, of their interactions by irresponsibility, self-indulgence, interpersonal intrusiveness, and social rule breaking. Lifestyle criminals appear to have similar thought patterns to early adolescents and, thus, have little conception of responsibility and self-discipline. The arrested development of the cognition process, regardless if constitutional or environmental, tends to set these individuals up for failure. This failure applies not only to criminal situations but also to the wide range of common situations, such as school, work and home.

Locating some eight "primitive cognitive characteristics," Walters and White examine the thinking patterns of lifestyle criminals and find that, from an early age, these individuals present chronic management problems. Because of their adolescent-like motives, lifestyle criminals rationalize their behavior and are preoccupied with short-term hedonism, which is destructive in the long run. Finally, Walters and White argue that lifestyle criminals direct their behavior toward "losing in dramatic and destructive ways" (1989a:8). In consistently choosing self-interested and hedonistic alternatives, criminals perpetuate their behavior. Although this perspective's recognition of psychological variables serves to introduce some complexity to the crime event, it is also true that complexity is lost with the lack of social factors. Moreover, the emphasis on a dominant cognitive variable yields a relatively static view of reality.

Social Control Theories

Michael Gottfredson and Travis Hirschi in a book (1990) that follows four prefatory articles (Hirschi and Gottfredson, 1983; Hirschi and Gottfredson, 1987; Gottfredson and Hirschi, 1989; Hirschi and Gottfredson, 1989) present a theory of crime based on an examination of both crime and criminality. Their work variously refers to this perspective as a "propensity-event" theory, a "general" theory and, finally, as a "low self-control" theory. The key ingredients are under-lying propensities (crime-proneness), early childhood socialization, and the conditions under which these translate into crime. Also of importance to the perspective is the fact that Gottfredson and Hirschi redefine crime so that they refer only to self-interested behaviors ("acts of force or fraud undertaken in the pursuit of self-interest" [1990:15]).

Certain traits manifest themselves among individuals, for example, aggressiveness, impulsivity, self-centeredness and intelligence.

Gottfredson and Hirschi argue that these traits are established early and persist throughout life. They view child-rearing practices as the prime influence on the formation of certain propensities, with inadequate child-rearing practices serving to produce directions conducive to criminality. These very traits are often associated with particular social settings and thus are difficult to separate from those settings. The relationship with crime is less than perfect because they are not necessary conditions for crime and, in fact, will reveal themselves in noncriminal activities as well. Those other activities, though, may share some of the characteristics of crime (e.g., alcohol or drug use). In short, Gottfredson and Hirschi assume that criminal traits are naturally present and "in the absence of socialization the child will tend to be high on crime potential" (1989:61).

Crime, on the other hand, is viewed as an event in time and space and several factors may need to be present for a crime to occur. If an individual has a pre-existing propensity toward crime, crime becomes attractive; thus, the crime-propensity affinity entices individuals and promises pleasure. The rationalist point of the theory proposes that the crime-event must be capable of gratifying the offender and that consequences (perceived or real) do not surmount the pleasure to be gained from the event. Of course, the event requires certain conditions, namely, that there be something upon which to perpetrate the event and that the situation suggests a lack of undesirable consequences. There may also be internal conditions (strength, speed, presence of alcohol) that assist in the evaluation of the event. The theory presumes that criminals have no special motivations; everyone is similarly motivated. The real problem is self-control. Low self-control yields a higher probability that an individual will engage in crime; high self-control yields a low probability for criminal behavior (1990:89).

The "general theory of crime" appears to be the most popular of current theories. At its base, the combination of propensity and event within one theory shows promise of understanding the contributions of various dimensions to the criminological event. The authors accept psychological, and even biological, evidence about individual differences in crime propensity. However, the major contribution of this perspective to complexity is the realization that there are many forms of behavior that are analogous to crime. The arguments in the book suggest, and even maintain, that other, similarly pleasurable behavioral events may substitute for crime. That is, crime is one of a group of similarly treated behaviors, any one of which is suitable as an outcome of the same grouping of causal variables. Thus, the authors recognize the potential for complexity in outcomes and, in essence, propose a multiple dependent variable. On the other hand, by retreating to a single dominant variable (early childhood socialization), the theory loses complexity and becomes a relative static approach to explaining crime over the life of an individual.

Subjective Theory

One of the most controversial and original theoretical positions of the 1980s is found in *Seductions of Crime: Moral and Sensual Attractions in Doing Evil* by Jack Katz (1988). Katz offers a critique of positivist criminology, largely by noting that many of those predicted to commit crime do not, while many of those who are not predicted to commit crime do so. In addition, he points out that those predicted to commit crime often do not for long periods of time, even though the background factors remain the same. His final critique, and the one most central, is that the standard background factors cannot predict which individuals will engage in crime.

Katz's theory revolves around the notion that the experiential foreground is crucial to the choice to engage in criminal action. Perhaps the term "choice" is not exactly correct here, because Katz means that certain things are viewed as seductive by the individual and are empowered to generate action. Different crimes have different forms of seduction, but they are all passionate, exciting, and relevant to the constructed identity of the offender. In a sense, crime is as Thrasher once described gang delinquency—it can be fun.

The essence of violent forms of crime is more than fun, in that the offender transcends normal life by becoming a "badass" or becoming tough, mean, and chaotic. By being unpredictable and chaotic the robber establishes himself or herself as beyond the normal experience and uses the threat of chaos to usurp the orderly lifestyle of victims. By being "alien" the badass generates a posture that shows more than abnormal morality, but in fact that he or she comes from a "morally alien place" (p. 88). In addition the actor becomes "hard" thereby refuting attempts of others at control and resisting social malleability. Thus, the individual creates "an angle of moral superiority over the intended victim" (p. 169) and the system at large. Where murder is concerned, the killer is moved from the "eternally humiliating situation" to passionate rage and, finally, a "righteous slaughter." The humiliation is not simply an attack on the individual, but it is an affront to an "eternal human value." Rage, then, is less unbridled than it is a focused effort to redeem oneself, generate power, and defend the eternal value. Thus the term "righteous slaughter" is used to denote that the murder has been undertaken as a last stand to correct a wrong. Similar observations are made about shoplifting and youth gangs.

Katz's phenomenological perspective requires that one understand the situation from the view of the offender. Without this focus, the offense appears irrational. The problem, of course, is that Katz not only has to understand and appreciate these offenses from the perspective of the offender, but that he also has to equate universality (or at least a lion's share) with this understanding. We do not know whether all offenders, most of them, or a few of them share in these meanings. The advantage of Katz's position is that it sensitizes criminologists to alternative meanings of deviance. Rationality for the actor can be vastly different from the imputed rationality of the observer. Moreover, this perspective has a rather spiritual flavor to the gains of crime. As a result, Katz's work has found rough ground in a criminological world that is largely objective and deterministic. It does, however, promise an exponential increase for criminological complexity, particularly if his subjective approach is *added* to the existing quantitative paradigm.

Conflict/Critical Theory

Square of Crime

One of the major criticisms of critical theory throughout the 1970s and 80s was that the perspective was not relevant to the lives of the powerless, i.e., those who lived in high crime areas and who were frequently victimized by street criminals. Recognizing the validity of the critique, some critical criminologists created a "left realist" perspective that expressly focused on what critical criminology could do for the public. In a theoretically sensitive version of left realism, Jock Young (1992) created what he referred to as the "square of crime." Four elements—victim, offender, state (formal control), and society (informal control)—come together to describe the interplay of forces dealing with the criminal event. Depending on the popularity of Young's work with critical criminologists, the perspective promises a richer, more complex picture of crime. Given the track record of most mainstream criminologists ignoring critical theory, however, that richness will probably fail to enter dominant theory.

Postmodern Theory

Postmodern theory is largely a product of the 1990s. While it is many things, recent work seems to focus on two major directions: the use of linguistic theory, or semiotics, and chaos-based theory. The semiotic version (see Milovanovic, 1997a, and Arrigo, 1996) trades primarily on the writings of Jacques Lacan (1981), introducing a reality formed by metaphors and linguistic concepts to the workings of the criminal justice system. These theorists note that the created reality is such that those accused of crime are inherently disadvantaged. This appreciation of the subjective reality of legal structures and concepts adds to an understanding of crime, particularly the structuring of responses to crime. As with most critical theory, however, there is little likelihood that mainstream criminology will see fit to incorporate its concepts.

Chaos-based postmodern theories (see Milovanovic, 1997b) are just beginning to emerge and, in one sense, show more promise of being reflected in mainstream criminology. This is primarily because chaos theories offer a radically different view of the world yet do not have the intellectual and conceptual baggage left over from radical/critical theory. As far as the conflict/consensus debate goes, chaos theories are relatively appositional. Another name for the perspective, at least from physics and related fields, is complexity theory. The general idea is that highly complex systems are difficult to model in a linear fashion, and the interaction of hundreds (perhaps millions) of variables makes static analysis virtually worthless. Thus, chaotic systems are nonlinear and dynamic representations of reality. In addition, there are no ideological positions that require variables from only one discipline (actually, multi-disciplinary models are common). The main problem with such theories is that traditional analytical techniques are virtually worthless, making the approach a challenge to the dominant analytical paradigm.

Feminist Theories

Perhaps mirroring the evolution of criminological theory, feminist theorists have now developed a typology of specialized perspectives (liberal, radical, Marxist, and socialist feminism). This development has been applied to criminology and attempts have been made to summarize existing criminological work into these perspectives (Daly and Chesney-Lind, 1988; Danner, 1989; Simpson, 1989).

Despite early enthusiasm for the hypothesis that there was a link between liberation and crime, meaningful research support never materialized. Simpson (1989) postulates that the quest may have even distracted researchers from more productive variables such as economics, class, and opportunities. While Simpson believes that liberal (more quantitative and more mainstream democratic/academic) contributions are now being answered with more radical critiques, she looks forward to work that emphasizes qualitative, historical, and subjectivist approaches. In the face of debate about the precise role of the feminist perspective, writers like Daly and Chesney-Lind (1988) call for integration of feminist thought in all areas of criminology. Socialist feminism in particular, Danner (1989) speculates, with its emphasis on the overlapping effects of class, race, and gender will serve to strengthen critical thought.

Power-Control Theory

One major approach appears to have heeded a call for combining critical and feminist thought. The work of John Hagan and colleagues (1989a, 1989b) can be considered the first major work in a "structural" perspective since the 1950s. Hagan meshes structural variations in crime rates with a version of stratification informed by neo-Marxist conflict theory. Rather than using the concept of class or income as measures of stratification, he uses power. In fact, here the argument is rather straightforward conflict theory: those with more power are less likely to be criminalized or punished and, conversely, actions against them are more likely to be viewed as serious. Where it diverges, however, is that the notion of degree of power is rejected for a version in which who controls whom is critical. Thus, a "command" status is derived for those who have freedom of activity, who control the activities of others, and who share the authority of society. This status also conveys that these individuals are relatively free from control themselves. An "obey" status is reserved for all those who are subordinate to such control.

Perhaps the main point of the Hagan approach is that a positive relationship is predicted between power and crime rather than the usual negative one. He does this by focusing on a larger version of "crime" than street crime, which of course is still associated with those in the "obey" status. White-collar crime and other expanded versions of crime, usually seen as non-crime, are the ones that most concern Hagan in making this prediction. The argument points out that "command" status carries with it the freedom from having one's activities associated with criminality; thus, the distribution of official crime rates is rather spurious to the issue of criminality. Crime rates are, however, critical to the issue of whose interests are threatened and who is processed by the authority structure of the criminal justice system.

Hagan's work carries on the tradition of structural conflict theories and is rather reminiscent of Weber's conceptions of power and authority. The extension of these ideas into an association with risk-taking and the learning of risk-taking behavior from one's parents makes this version unique, however. Similarly, the incorporation of gender is valuable. Hagan argues that power relationships in larger society, especially in the workplace, are reflected in the family. In short, the relationships one learns in the work world, the methods of establishing authority and dominance over others, are carried home to the family. Members of different social classes experience different power relationships and construct different family relationships. Similarly, because the workplace relationships vary by gender, males and females experience different roles, expectations and values. The combination of social class and gender experiences creates structured family relationships that help to explain the social distribution of delinquency. The more patriarchal the family structure, the greater is the gender gap in delinquent behavior between sons and daughters. On the other hand, a more egalitarian family will reproduce relations that lead to sons and daughters participating more equally in delinquency.

Strain Theory

The best known of contemporary versions of strain theory is one created by Robert Agnew (1985, 1989, 1992): general strain theory. Agnew contends that traditional strain theories look at positively valued goals. He asserts that another ingredient should be added: the avoidance of painful (or negative) situations. Just as an individual's goals can be blocked, so can the ability to avoid undesirable things or stressful life events. For instance, a juvenile may not be able to avoid a bad family situation, may drop out of school as a solution to poor grades, or even hide from peer rejection. All of these things may yield levels of frustration as high as those from blocked aspirations or immediate goals. When both positive blockage and negative avoidance are combined, the stress levels suggest that we can expect the highest rates of delinquency or deviance.

A second contemporary adaptation of strain theories is that of Steven Messner and Richard Rosenfeld (1994). Given the traditional Mertonian scheme that economic sources of strain yield anomic conditions, they argue that an entire level of non-economic institutions has been omitted. A more rounded picture of structural constraints on deviance include the contributions of such institutions as the family, schools, religion and law. For anomie to work, not only is a disjunction of goals and means necessary, but social institutions must also be weakened. They posit that a dysjunction affects these institutions in such a way as to contribute to a loss of control, i.e., an anomic environment weakens the family's control over its members and thus its power to curtail deviant behavior. The theory obviously incorporates concepts from control theory and provides a bridge from cultural controls (old strain versions) to more personal levels of control.

Both of these additions to the Mertonian strain approach provide another level of explanation to the structural variables of the original perspective and demonstrate the value of relationships between cultural strain and personal factors. This acknowledgment of the complexity of strain is an important advance in combining structural factors with the individual-level variables. Nonetheless, the theories still fail to treat factors that are outside the traditional offender environment and remain preeminently sociological. In addition, while there are some implications for dynamic relationships, the theories primarily yield a static view of reality.

Metatheory, Integrated Theory, and Interdisciplinary Theory

Metatheory

Criminology, as with sociology in general, has expressed mild interest in metatheory. In general, metatheory concerns itself with the organization of principles that can be used to make sense of theories. Metatheory is not directly testable and, for that reason, is eschewed by some (Gibbs, 1989). It does, however, have its uses, particularly in the identification of levels of explanation of various theories (Short, 1989). Unless theoretical assumptions and points of focus are clearly identified, there is little to prevent improper tests and integration of those theories. Some of those theories, for instance, treat either crime or criminal behavior, two rather divergent foci that are often treated as if they were identical. Some writers, for example Joan McCord (1989), also view meta-theories as approaches that meld together existing theories. Her concern, however, is that we may simply integrate theories without having criteria against which to measure the adequacy of our theories. Integrative theorizing, however, appears to be in vogue. One document of this trend (Messner, Krohn and Liska, 1989) reported on papers presented at a 1987 conference on theoretical integration. Authors of these various papers represent most of the major criminological theoreticians and discuss micro-level, macro-level, and cross-level integration. On the whole, there are some insights (Akers, 1989; Bursik, 1989; Bernard, 1989; Hagan, 1989b; Tittle, 1989), but the consensus argument across the papers is there are too many problems for successful integration to take place (see especially the essays by Hirschi, 1989; Gibbs, 1989; Giordano, 1989; Meier, 1989; Short, 1989; Swigert, 1989; and Thornberry, 1989). Notwithstanding this consensus, there are some interesting integrative and integrated theories that were developed in the late 1980s and 1990s.

Integrative Shaming

The most coherent, and novel, recent integrated theory has been presented by John Braithwaite (1989b, 1989c). He incorporates opportunity, subcultural, control, social learning, and labeling theories to produce a theory which relies on the notion of differential shaming. Beginning with opportunity theory, Braithwaite notes there are aspirations and means, both legitimate and illegitimate. For criminality or delinquency to occur, blocked legitimate opportunities must be replaced by available illegitimate ones. Subcultural theories add the concept of organization for learning and transmission of law-breaking values. Here, Braithwaite notes the contrast with social control theory: one creates conformity with the law, while the other creates conformity with the subculture and nonconformity with the law. The direction to be taken remains problematic; a "tipping point" is needed.

Differential shaming is posited as that tipping point. The diverse forms of shaming are available both to conventional and subcultural groups. To the extent that an offender is exposed to shaming or anticipates shaming, a tipping point is reached. Two forms of shaming are also presented: disintegrative shaming and integrative shaming. The former fails to reconcile a shamed offender with the community or subgroup, thus resulting in an outcast status and greater deviance. The latter reaccepts the shamed offender with reconciliatory gestures and separates the evil act from the character of the offender. The obvious policy implications are that acts can be strongly sanctioned, but a reformed offender can be treated in a forgiving fashion. Since subcultures have power to shame as well as the moral order, the theoretical problem is to overcome the subcultural effect by a network of communities operating under a reintegrative shaming modality. Braithwaite's article on organizational crime (1989c) makes just such an attempt and a subsequent article (1991) enlarges the perspective.

Braithwaite's interesting attempt at integration has been noted (see Gibbons, 1994) but remains on the periphery of popular theory. In some ways this is unfortunate because it is not only the most coherent of integrative theories but it is also the most adaptive. At the least the book, and the attention paid to it, is indicative of an ongoing interest in theoretical integration.

Interdisciplinary Theory

Where interdisciplinary theories are concerned, one of the major psychology of crime theorists, Hans Eysenck, reappeared with a new book (Eysenck and Gudjonnson, 1989) entitled *The Causes and Cures of Criminality*. An article in the first volume of *Advances in Criminological Theory*, however, constitutes an easily-read review of Eysenck's main ideas (Eysenck, 1989). Criticizing sociological criminology, Eysenck found two main faults: (1) Social causes are secondary to psychological causes because social factors must act through individuals and (2) improvements in the conditions of such sociological mainstays of poverty, inequality, and bad housing lead to positive correlations with crime, not negative ones. In addition, he adds that scientific theories are faddish and that rejection of psychological causation is premature and largely unfounded. Andrews and Wormith (1989) make a similar assessment. They point out that the vested interests of sociological criminologists have created an "antipersonality" orientation that leads to a systematic rejection of individual differences in criminal propensity.

Eysenck's main theoretical position hinges around three major personality dimensions: psychoticism, extroversion, and neuroticism. Criminality generally is correlated with high degrees of all three, although certain types of crime may be correlated differently. Where

age is concerned, the younger offender is more likely to have high
levels of extroversion than neuroticism. Older offenders, on the other
hand, exhibit higher levels of neuroticism. In all age groups,
psychoticism is always important. Eysenck documents these relationships across various studies and countries and notes that "anti-social"
traits (smoking, legal or illegal drug use) are correlated with these
personality traits as well as criminality.

C. Ray Jeffery, as part of a series of writings, proffered an
interdisciplinary theory of criminal behavior in *Advances in
Criminological Theory* (1989a) and a criminology text (1989b). His
perspective is that sociological, psychological, and biological
characteristics interact in a systems model to produce criminal
behavior. He posits that individuals are born with particular biological
(genetic) and psychological characteristics that not only may predispose
but may actually cause certain forms of behavior. This "nature" is
independent of the socialization process present in the social
environment. There is, however, a good deal of interplay between
nature and nurture through physical environments and the feedback
mechanisms that exist in biochemical systems. For example, Jeffery
notes that poverty translates to a certain type of diet and exposure to
pollutants which is transformed by the biochemical system into
neurochemical compounds within the brain. Thus, poverty indirectly
leads to behavioral differences (and, potentially, criminal behavior)
through the interaction of individual and environment.

Jeffery is clearly suggesting that any theory of criminal behavior is
incomplete without a consideration of all elements that make up the
human organism. In addition, he also notes that a study of criminal
behavior is not possible without an understanding and theory of
criminal law. A summary of his overall approach that combines both
behavior and law is as follows: Humans are born with biological and
psychological differences. These differences lead to direct conflict with
other humans. In order to reduce this conflict, humans must be
socialized into conformity and, lacking this, control systems (the state
and criminal law) must be created to restrict behavior. Criminal
behavior is behavior thus restricted.

While Eysenck and Jeffery are not entirely compatible in their
respective approaches to interdisciplinary theory, there are, nonetheless,
some similarities. Both charge that sociological theories of crime and
criminal behavior overlook major individual factors. Both note that the
individual's makeup creates propensities and tendencies toward certain

behaviors. And both believe that any understanding o f behavior i s contingent on the interaction o f individuals with the environment. Unfortunately, the direction of criminology and criminal justice has been toward specialization. While they may be correct in calling for a more interdisciplinary approach to criminological problems, the field is likely to continue in its pursuit of the opposite direction. Their approaches suggest that criminologists would do well to incorporate the findings of other disciplines into an understanding of crime and the criminal event.

Life-Course Theory

In a new look at an old dataset, Robert Sampson and John Laub (1990, 1992, 1993) have noted that change over time is a critical component in explaining crime: the criminal experience is a dynamic one. Analyzing the Gluecks' (1950) old data on 1000 juveniles followed until age thirty-two, they found that traditional delinquency experiences predicted criminality in adult life. However, informal social control seemed to have an effect on the likelihood of delinquent experiences, and events after becoming an adult, such as job stability, were important in decreasing adult criminality. In other words, various forms of social bonds (particularly work, education, and the family) change the life trajectory of crime (1990:618) and at different points in life have differential effects. Just as they serve to reduce criminal activity, these bonds can also be broken and then act as a destabilizing force over the affected portion of the life course.

These findings and Sampson and Laub's theory of social control and "turning points" point to a useful dimension of criminal behavior for criminologists. The added complexity of examining a dynamic model of behavior provides a sensitivity to a potential "build-up" of factors that ultimately result in a "tipping-point" for behavior. Moreover, Sampson and Laub show other indications of appreciating of the depth and intricacy of the entire criminal event, for instance, as they briefly discuss the interaction of social reaction and age (1993:253).

Evolutionary Ecology Theory

The title of "the most complex theory" in recent theorizing belongs to Lawrence Cohen and Richard Machalek's evolutionary ecology perspective (with contributions by Bryan Vila [1994]). Ignoring the problem of crime committed by truly deviant individuals, they examine crime committed by otherwise normal people. The theory is drawn primarily from concepts in the fields of behavioral ecology and evolutionary biology and focuses on the diversity of "behavioral strategies" derived from social and personal interactions. The factors that contribute to criminality are variously sociocultural, constitutional, developmental, environmental, situational (opportunities), and psychological. If this perspective gains in popularity, it will clearly create a new paradigm by which we view reality. For this reason alone, it will probably be relegated to the sidewaters of criminological theory.

CONCLUSIONS

The relative theoretical quiet represented by the 1970s may have been the stultifying end of a paradigm (Kuhn, 1970). Buoyed by new evidence produced by environmental design and topographical research, some criminologists began to conceive of criminals as rational individuals who made their own behavioral choices from a patchwork of opportunity. Others, informed by advances in feminist thought, used age-old evidence on male/female crime to create gender-based explanations of socialization, power, and lifestyle differentials as they affect criminality. Yet others, tired of the orderly way in which mainstream theories relegated deviance to objective existence, insisted that crime is best understood as a subjective experience, a "seduction into evil" (Katz, 1988). Finally, some attempted to find new ways to reconstruct the old versions of criminological theories (Braithwaite, 1989b, 1991; Bursik, 1988, 1989; Cullen, 1984; Farnworth and Leiber, 1989; Hagan, 1989a, 1989b; Link *et al.* 1989; Luckenbill and Doyle, 1989; Paternoster and Iovanni, 1989), and work on deterrence became more sophisticated (Paternoster, 1989a, 1989b).

While the Kuhnian paradigm concept may not quite describe the happenings at the end of this decade (some argue that it simply does not fit the social sciences at all), it is reasonable to use it as a way of analyzing the experience. The emergence of a single paradigm has always been problematic in criminology, yet reference to "mainstream" criminology is common. This mainstream criminology, whatever form it may take, has largely been consensus based and, through the 1950s and 1960s, was some combination of structural-functionalist and Chicago School thought. Arguably, these mainstream theories at least had social determinism in common. The 1960s brought new forms of social determinist theories such as labeling, conflict, social learning, and social control, all of which (except radical versions of conflict) became mainstream criminology by the 1980s.

Perhaps because of the massive effort to test theory, the 1980s produced a period of doubt. No one theory seemed to hold up very well to evidence, although some were declared to be superior to others. Thus, some degree of consternation set in. If we borrow from Kuhn, the period was one of crisis. Criminology was not sure if it was to explain crime, criminal behavior, or some subset of crime; in fact, criminologists were not even sure if they had the right questions (Farrington, Ohlin and Wilson, 1986), let alone the right answers. The literature and research of the 1980s reflected this problem as well as a search for new directions.

While nothing like Kuhn's revolutionary phase has been reached, turmoil in the form of new theoretical insights in the late 1980s and 1990s has clearly begun to challenge the old paradigm of social determinism. The assumption of rationalism and the return of "natural propensities" allow the introduction of psychological and biological concepts into the explanation of criminality. At the same time, traditional notions of socially-structured crime conditions can be interpreted to mean there are persistent patterns of rationality, personality traits, or biological properties. Thus, the older perspectives do not necessarily die out; instead, they may be reworked to mesh with the new ideas.

Contemporary criminology, as the review in this chapter exhibits, is now fermenting nicely. Theorists are entertaining new evidence on criminality, while at the same time reconceptualizing and reassessing old evidence. The appreciation of complexity is perhaps a bit less clear. Some of the newer theories have added new dimensions to old pictures of crime yet, just as frequently, other theories have retreated to simplicity. The lessons of labeling and conflict have largely been ignored. When a new dimension is added, it seems that the entire focus is on that dimension instead of on the way multiple dimensions relate to the criminal event. For instance, the social reaction dimension of labeling largely failed to get criminologists to *add* that dimension to existing offender dimensions and the newer victim dimension of routine activities theories has similarly failed to enlarge theory.

While there may be some doubt about the likelihood of an appreciation of a more complex criminological reality, what is clear is that new ideas are now afoot. The direction of these new ideas, however, is not yet clear because of a diversity of perspectives.

Nonetheless, the field is seemingly on the verge of a paradigm revolution as energetic and far-reaching as the labeling and conflict-oriented movements of the early 1960s.

NOTES

1. I apologize to those who have made contributions to criminological theory and have been omitted here. The fact of expediency does not suggest a lack of contribution.

2. Mayhew et al. (1976) in England were developing a similar rational choice model referred to as an "opportunity perspective."

3. The criminal personality theory of Yochelson and Samenow (1976) also belonged to the period, but criminologists were still sociologically oriented enough to want a more social perspective and, theoretically, criminal personality had little impact. Governmental figures, on the other hand, embraced the perspective.

4. Marilyn McShane made substantial contributions to this section.

REFERENCES

Adler, Freda (1975). *Sisters in Crime: The Rise of the New Female Criminal.* New York, NY: McGraw-Hill.

Agnew, Robert (1985). A revised strain theory of delinquency. *Social Forces* 64: 151–167.

Agnew, Robert (1989). A longitudinal test of the revised strain theory. *Journal of Quantitative Criminology* 5: 373–387.

Agnew, Robert (1992). Foundation for a general strain theory of crime and delinquency. *Criminology* 30: 47–88.

Agnew, Robert and Helene R. White (1992). An empirical test of general strain theory. *Criminology* 30: 475–500.

Akers, Ronald L. (1973). *Deviant Behavior: A Social Learning Approach.* Belmont, CA: Wadsworth.

Akers, Ronald L. (1989). A social behaviorist's perspective on integration of theories of crime and deviance. Pp. 23–36 in Steven F. Messner, Marvin D. Krohn and Allen E. Liska (eds.) *Theoretical Integration in the Study of Deviance and Crime: Problems and Prospects.* Albany, NY: State University of New York Press.

Andrews, D.A., and J. Stephen Wormith (1989). Personality and crime: Knowledge destruction and construction in criminology. *Justice Quarterly* 6: 289–309.

Arrigo, Bruce (1996). *The Contours of Psychiatric Justice: A Postmodern Critique of Mental Illness, Criminal Insanity and the Law.* New York, NY: Garland.

Bernard, Thomas J. (1989). A theoretical approach to integration. Pp. 137–159 in Steven F. Messner, Marvin D. Krohn, and Allen E. Liska (eds.) *Theoretical Integration in the Study of Deviance and Crime: Problems and Prospects.* Albany, NY: State University of New York Press.

Braithwaite, John (1989a). The state of criminology: Theoretical decay or renaissance? *Australian and New Zealand Journal of Criminology,* 22: 129–135.

Braithwaite, John (1989b). *Crime, Shame, and Reintegration.* Cambridge, UK: Cambridge University Press.

Braithwaite, John (1989c). Criminological theory and organizational crime. *Criminology* 6: 333–358.

Braithwaite, John (1991). Poverty, power, white-collar crime and the paradoxes of criminological theory. *Australian and New Zealand Journal of Criminology* 24: 40–58.

Burgess, Robert L., and Ronald L. Akers (1966). A differential association-reinforcement theory of criminal behavior. *Social Problems* 14: 128–147.

Bursik, Robert J., Jr. (1988). Social disorganization and theories of crime and delinquency. *Criminology* 26: 519–545.

Bursik, Robert J., Jr. (1989). Political decision-making and ecological models of delinquency: Conflict and consensus. Pp. 105–117 in Steven F. Messner, Marvin D. Krohn, and Allen E. Liska (eds.), *Theoretical Integration in the Study of Deviance and Crime: Problems and Prospects.* Albany, NY: State University of New York Press.

Chambliss, William J. (1975). Toward a political economy of crime. *Theory and Society* 2: 149–169.

Clarke, Ronald V., and Derek B. Cornish (1985). Modeling offenders' decisions: A framework for research and policy. Pp. 147–185 in Michael Tonry and Norval Morris (eds.) *Crime and Justice: An Annual Review of Research,* vol. 6. Chicago, IL: University of Chicago Press.

Cohen, Lawrence E., and Marcus Felson (1979). Social change and crime rate trends: A routine activities approach. *American Sociological Review* 44: 588–607.

Cohen, Lawrence E., and Richard Machalek (1988). A general theory of expropriative crime: An evolutionary ecological approach. *American Journal of Sociology* 94: 465–501.

Cornish, Derek B., and Ronald V. Clarke (eds) (1986). *The Reasoning Criminal: Rational Choice Perspectives on Offending.* New York, NY: Springer-Verlag.

Cullen, Francis T. (1984). *Rethinking Crime and Deviance Theory: The Emergence of a Structuring Tradition.* Totowa, NJ: Rowman and Allanheld.

Daly, Kathleen, and Meda Chesney-Lind (1988). Feminism and criminology. *Justice Quarterly* 5: 497–538.

Danner, Mona (1989). Socialist feminism: A brief introduction. *Critical Criminologist* 1: 1–2.

Elliott, Delbert, David Huizinga, and Suzanne Ageton (1985). *Explaining Delinquency and Drug Use.* Beverly Hills, CA: Sage.

Eysenck, Hans J. (1989). Personality and Criminality: A Dispositional Analysis. Pp. 89–110 in William S. Laufer and Freda Adler (eds.) *Advances in Criminological Theory,* vol. 1. New Brunswick, NJ: Transaction.

Eysenck, Hans J., and I. Gudjonnson (1989). *The Causes and Cures of Criminality.* New York, NY: Plenum Press.

Farnworth, Margaret, and Michael Leiber (1989). Strain theory revisited: Economic goals, educational means and delinquency. *American Sociological Review* 54: 263–274.

Farrington, David P., Lloyd E. Ohlin and James Q. Wilson (1986). *Understanding and Controlling Crime.* New York, NY: Springer-Verlag.

Gibbons, Don C. (1994). *Talking about Crime and Criminals: Problems and Issues in Theory Development in Criminology.* Englewood Cliffs, NJ: Prentice Hall.

Gibbs, Jack P. (1989). Three perennial issues in the sociology of deviance. Pp. 179–198 in Steven F. Messner, Marvin D. Krohn, and Allen E. Liska (eds.) *Theoretical Integration in the Study of Deviance and Crime: Problems and Prospects.* Albany, NY: State University of New York Press.

Giordano, Peggy C. (1989). Confronting control theory's negative cases. Pp. 261–278 in Steven F. Messner, Marvin D. Krohn, and Allen E. Liska (eds.) *Theoretical Integration in the Study of Deviance and Crime: Problems and Prospects.* Albany, NY: State University of New York Press.

Glueck, Sheldon and Eleanor (1950). *Unraveling Juvenile Delinquency.* New York, NY: The Commonwealth Fund.

Gordon, David (1973). Capitalism, class and crime in America. *Crime and Delinquency* 19: 163–186.

Gottfredson, Michael, and Travis Hirschi (1989). A propensity-event theory of crime. Pp. 57–67 in William S. Laufer and Freda Adler (eds.) *Advances in Criminological Theory*, vol. 1. New Brunswick, NJ: Transaction.

Gottfredson, Michael, and Travis Hirschi (1990). *A General Theory of Crime*. Stanford, CA: Stanford University Press.

Grasmick, Harold G., and Robert J. Bursik (1990). Conscience, significant others, and rational choice: Extending the deterrence model. *Law and Society Review* 24: 837–862.

Grasmick, Harold G. and Donald E. Green (1980). Legal punishment, social disapproval, and internalization as inhibitors of illegal behavior. *Journal of Criminal Law and Criminology* 71: 325–335.

Green, Donald E. (1989) Measures of illegal behavior in individual-level research. *Journal of Research in Crime and Delinquency* 26: 253–275.

Hagan, John (1989a). *Structural Criminology*. New Brunswick, NJ: Rutgers University Press.

Hagan, John (1989b). Micro- and macro-structures of delinquency causation and a power-control theory of gender and delinquency. Pp. 213–227 in Steven F. Messner, Marvin D. Krohn and Allen E. Liska (eds.) *Theoretical Integration in the Study of Deviance and Crime: Problems and Prospects*. Albany, NY: State University of New York Press.

Hindelang, Michael J., Michael Gottfredson and James Garofalo (1978). *Victims of Personal Crime: An Empirical Foundation for a Theory of Personal Victimization*. Cambridge, MA: Ballinger.

Hirschi, Travis (1969). *Causes of Delinquency*. Berkeley, CA: University of California Press.

Hirschi, Travis (1989). Exploring alternatives to integrated theory. Pp. 37–49 in Steven F. Messner, Marvin D. Krohn, and Allen E. Liska (eds.) *Theoretical Integration in the Study of Deviance and Crime: Problems and Prospects*. Albany, NY: State University of New York Press.

Hirschi, Travis, and Michael Gottfredson (1983). Age and the explanation of crime. *American Journal of Sociology* 89: 522–584.

Hirschi, Travis, and Michael Gottfredson (1987). Causes of white-collar crime. *Criminology* 25: 949–974.

Hirschi, Travis, and Michael Gottfredson (1989). The significance of white-collar crime for a general theory of crime. *Criminology* 27: 359–371.

Jeffery, C. Ray (1971). *Crime Prevention Through Environmental Design*. Beverly Hills, CA: Sage.

Jeffery, C. Ray (1989a). An interdisciplinary theory of criminal behavior. Pp. 69–87 in William S. Laufer and Freda Adler (eds.) *Advances in Criminological Theory*, vol. 1. New Brunswick, NJ: Transaction.

Jeffery, C. Ray (1989b). *Criminology: An Interdisciplinary Approach.* Englewood Cliffs, NJ: Prentice Hall.

Katz, Jack (1988). *Seductions of Crime: Moral and Sensual Attractions in Doing Evil.* New York, NY: Basic Books.

Kuhn, Thomas (1970). *The Structure of Scientific Revolutions,* 2nd ed. Chicago: University of Chicago Press.

Lacan, Jacques (1981). *The Four Fundamental Concepts of Psycho-Analysis.* New York, NY: Norton.

Link, Bruce, Francis T. Cullen, Elmer Struening, Patrick E. Shrout and Bruce P. Dohrewend (1989). A modified labeling theory approach to mental disorders: An empirical assessment. *American Sociological Review* 54: 400–423.

Luckenbill, David F., and Daniel P. Doyle (1989). Structural position and violence: Developing a cultural explanation. *Criminology* 27: 419–433.

Mayhew, Pat M., Ronald V. Clarke, A. Sturman, and J.M. Hough (1976). *Crime as Opportunity.* Home Office Research Study no. 24. London, UK: H.M. Stationery Office.

McCord, Joan (1989). Theory, pseudotheory, and metatheory. Pp. 127–145 in William S. Laufer and Freda Adler (eds.) *Advances in Criminological Theory,* vol. 1. New Brunswick, NJ: Transaction.

Meier, Robert F. (ed.) (1985). *Theoretical Methods in Criminology.* Beverly Hills, CA: Sage.

Meier, Robert F. (1989). Deviance and differentiation. Pp. 199–212 in Steven F. Messner, Marvin D. Krohn, and Alan A. Liska (eds.) *Theoretical Integration in the Study of Deviance and Crime: Problems and Prospects.* Albany, NY: State University of New York Press.

Meier, Robert F., and Weldon T. Johnson (1977). Deterrence as social control: The legal and extralegal production of conformity. *American Sociological Review* 42: 292–304.

Messner, Steven F., Marvin D. Krohn, and Alan A. Liska (eds.) (1989). *Theoretical Integration in the Study of Deviance and Crime: Problems and Prospects.* Albany, NY: State University of New York Press.

Messner, Steven F., and Richard Rosenfeld (1994). *Crime and the American Dream.* Belmont, CA: Wadsworth.

Milovanovic, Dragan (1997a). *Postmodern Criminology.* New York, NY: Garland.

Milovanovic, Dragan (ed.) (1997b). *Chaos, Criminology and Social Justice: The New Orderly (Dis)Order.* Westport, CT: Praeger.

Minor, W. William (1977). A deterrence-control theory of crime. Pp. 117–137 in Robert F. Meier (ed.) *Theory in Criminology: Contemporary Views.* Beverly Hills, CA: Sage.

Nagin, Daniel S., and Raymond Paternoster (1991). Preventive effects of the perceived risk of arrest: Testing an expanded conception of deterrence. *Criminology* 29: 561–585.

Paternoster, Raymond (1989a). Absolute and restrictive deterrence in a panel of youth: Explaining the onset, persistence/desistence and frequency of delinquent offending. *Social Problems* 36: 289–308.

Paternoster, Raymond (1989b). Decisions to participate in and desist from four types of common delinquency: Deterrence and the rational choice perspective. *Law and Society Review* 23: 7–40.

Paternoster, Raymond, and Lee Iovanni (1989). The labeling perspective and delinquency: An elaboration of the theory and assessment of the evidence. *Justice Quarterly* 6: 359–394

Paternoster, Raymond, Linda E. Saltzman, Gordon P. Waldo, and Theodore G. Chiricos (1983). Perceived risk and social control: Do sanctions really deter? *Law and Society Review* 17: 457–480.

Paternoster, Raymond, and Ruth Triplett (1988). Disaggregating self-reported delinquency and its implications for theory. *Criminology* 26: 591–615.

Quinney, Richard (1970). *The Social Reality of Crime.* Boston, MA: Little, Brown.

Quinney, Richard (1974). *Critique of Legal Order.* Boston, MA: Little, Brown.

Quinney, Richard (1977). *Class, State, and Crime: On the Theory and Practice of Criminal Justice.* New York, NY: McKay.

Sampson, Robert J., and John H. Laub (1990). Crime and deviance over the life course: The salience of adult social bonds. *American Sociological Review* 55:609–627.

Sampson, Robert J., and John H. Laub (1992). Crime and deviance in the life course. *Annual Review of Sociology* 18: 63–84.

Sampson, Robert J., and John H. Laub (1993). *Crime in the Making: Pathways and Turning Points Through Life.* Cambridge, MA: Harvard University Press.

Schwendinger, Herman and Julia (1985). *Adolescent Subcultures and Delinquency.* New York, NY: Praeger.

Shearing, Clifford (1989). Decriminalizing criminology: Reflections on the literal and tropological meaning of the term. *Canadian Journal of Criminology* 31: 169–178.

Short, J. F., Jr. (1985). The level of explanation problem in criminology. Pp. 51–72 in Robert F. Meier (ed.) *Theoretical Methods in Criminology*. Beverly Hills, CA: Sage, 1985.

Short, James F., Jr.(1989). Exploring integration of theoretical levels of explanation: Notes on gang delinquency. Pp. 243–259 in Steven F. Messner, Marvin D. Krohn, and Allen E. Liska (eds.) *Theoretical Integration in the Study of Deviance and Crime: Problems and Prospects*. Albany, NY: State University of New York Press.

Simon, Rita J. (1976). *Women and Crime*. Lexington, MA: Lexington Books.

Simpson, Sally (1989). Feminist theory, crime and justice. *Criminology* 27: 605–625.

Spitzer, Steven (1975). Toward a Marxian theory of deviance. *Social Problems* 22: 638–651.

Swigert, Victoria L. (1989). The discipline as data: Resolving the theoretical crisis in criminology. Pp. 129–135 in Steven F. Messner, Marvin D. Krohn, and Allen E. Liska (eds.) *Theoretical Integration in the Study of Deviance and Crime: Problems and Prospects*. Albany, NY: State University of New York Press.

Taylor, Ian, Paul Walton, and Jock Young (1973). *The New Criminology: For a Social Theory of Deviance*. London, UK: Routledge and Kegan Paul.

Thornberry, Terence P. (1989). Reflections on the advantages and disadvantages of theoretical integration. Pp. 51–60 in Steven F. Messner, Marvin D. Krohn and Allen E. Liska (eds.) *Theoretical Integration in the Study of Deviance and Crime: Problems and Prospects*. Albany, NY: State University of New York Press.

Tifft, Larry (1979). The coming redefinitions of crime: An anarchist perspective. *Social Problems* 26: 392–402.

Tittle, Charles R. (1989). Prospects for synthetic theory: A consideration of macro-level criminological activity. Pp. 161–178 in Steven F. Messner, Marvin D. Krohn, and Allen E. Liska (eds.) *Theoretical Integration in the Study of Deviance and Crime: Problems and Prospects*. Albany, NY: State University of New York Press.

Tittle, Charles R. (1985).The assumption that general theories are not possible. Pp. 93–121 in Robert F. Meier (ed.) *Theoretical Methods in Criminology*. Beverly Hills, CA: Sage.

Tunnell, Kenneth D. (1992). *Choosing Crime: The Criminal Calculus of Property Offenders*. Chicago, IL: Nelson-Hall.

Vila, Bryan (1994). A general paradigm for understanding criminal behavior: Extending evolutionary ecological theory. *Criminology* 32: 311–360.

Walters, Glenn D. (1990). *The Criminal Lifestyle*. Beverly Hills, CA: Sage.

Walters, Glenn D. (1989). Putting more thought into criminology. *International Journal of Offender Therapy and Comparative Criminology* 30: v–vii.

Walters, Glenn D., and Thomas W. White (1989a). The thinking criminal: A cognitive model of lifestyle criminality. *Criminal Justice Research Bulletin* 4(4): 1–10.

Walters, Glenn D., and Thomas W. White (1989b). Heredity and crime: Bad genes or bad research. *Criminology* 27: 455–481.

Whitehead, John T. (1986). The criminological imagination: Another view. *Criminal Justice Review* 10: 22–26.

Williams, Frank P., III (1984). The demise of the criminological imagination: A critique of recent criminology. *Justice Quarterly* 1: 91–106.

Williams, Frank P., III (1985). Deterrence and social control: Rethinking the relationship. *Journal of Criminal Justice* 13: 141–151.

Williams, Kirk R., and Richard Hawkins (1989). The meaning of arrest for wife assault. *Criminology* 27: 163–181.

Wilson, James Q. (1975). *Thinking About Crime*. New York, NY: Basic Books.

Wilson, James Q., and Richard Herrnstein (1985). *Crime and Human Nature*. New York, NY: Simon and Schuster.

Yochelson, Samuel, and Stanton E. Samenow (1976). *The Criminal Personality*, vol 1., *A Profile for Change*. New York, NY: Jason Aronson.

Young, Jock (1992). Ten points of realism. Pp. 24–68 in Jock Young and Roger Matthews (eds.) *Rethinking Criminology: The Realist Debate*. London, UK: Sage.

CHAPTER THREE

A Critique of Contemporary Criminological Theory

INTRODUCTION

Theoretical constructions in criminology have had problems for quite some time. Some have argued that the reason has been a lack of testability in the theoretical statements (Gibbs, 1972), a lack of specificity (Gibbons, 1994), a paralysis (Wellford, 1989), or even a lack of imagination (Williams, 1984). In general, one could argue that most of the "new" concepts and ideas are contained in basic perspectives of the past. Certainly theorists have dealt with new variables, but these are usually novel measurement approaches to the same concepts. A close examination of the review in the previous chapter will lend credence to an "old becomes new" hypothesis. New perspectives have, indeed, appeared (labeling, radical theories, power-control theory), but it seems to me that after they show initial promise, mainstream criminology rejects them, or acknowledges and sets them aside, and returns to the same old approaches—with a traditional sociological focus on why people become criminal. Even within the traditional perspective, some new theories are accepted but most are not. If all acceptances and rejections were due to evidence, there would be no problem with this state of affairs. Unfortunately, this does not seem to be the case. There are other, equally viable, reasons for the rise and fall of theories, among them the form of background assumptions in theory, competition and levels of explanation, theoretical fashions and fads, emerging paradigms, reputation of theorists, and even perhaps the fact that when a quantitative "feeding frenzy" ends, a new approach is necessary to keep publication going.[1] This chapter will explore the most basic of these rationales for the popularity of theory.

INTERPRETING THEORY

Theorists rarely explain the background of the theories they develop. As a result, the values and assumptions behind the written works are left implicit. Indeed, there is sometimes much speculation about the "true" domain assumptions for the theory. Others, drawn to a theory for various reasons, are left to impute that background. When they do, the tendency to do so is based on their own values and the social situation of the moment.

Retrospective Interpretation and Theories

This has important implications for theory because it suggests that the *meaning* of a theory can be governed by interpretations of others. In fact, I wish to argue that the meaning of any theory is largely dictated by the current value set of scholars—theory becomes popularly reinterpreted.[2] The theory itself does not change, but what it means to the field does (in a sublime turn of phrase, postmodernists refer to this as the "death of the author"). Unless one is aware of this, theories and their histories can become reinterpreted to fit existing conceptions.

Why is this important? Borrowing a phrase from Erving Goffman (1959), this is theoretical *retrospective interpretation.* "Old" theory can be endowed with assumptions which never existed. Because of new and different interests at various points of time, any look back at an older theory is not an innocent one: The current interests and concerns themselves color the way in which the older theory is viewed. For example, after the field was deeply into self-report methodology and busy proposing theories based on that evidence, it became difficult to "see" the theoretical perspectives of the Chicago School as they were when originally proposed. Even more recently, an argument has developed over what Sutherland assumed in his differential association theory and Merton with his anomie theory.[3] The focus is not so much what Sutherland *actually* assumed but how it should be interpreted. Moreover, I will now argue that it is not interpretation but *reinterpretation* that the argument is over.

The Necessity of Reinterpretation

Why should reinterpretation take place? Every new perspective needs to show that it is "better" than the old, and the easiest way to do this is to reconstruct a negative version of the old theory using the perspective and language of the new one, thereby decreasing its popularity. One might be moved to charge "new" theorists with purposefully distorting older theories. This is not what I mean to convey here, however, because no malicious intent is required. Instead, the problem is more likely one of differing views of social reality. What should be kept in mind is that supporters of the new are seeing social reality in a different way from the old—a view that was never possible for the original theorists. The new view is a product of social time and place, i.e., the context of social life. I believe new social realities lead to a relatively common, and unintentional, process of discrediting older theory in favor of newer theory. That which they have "always been" is something they never were—theories are reborn.

Reconstruction of Domain Assumptions

The rationale for these comments on reinterpretation lies primarily with Alvin Gouldner's (1970) work on domain assumptions which served to precipitate discussion on the unstated assumptions behind many theoretical perspectives. A classic example, which predates Gouldner's work, is Jack Gibbs' (1966) discussion of the "old and the new" conceptions of deviance—an essay derived from the social reality precipitated by labeling and an emerging conflict theory. In that essay, Gibbs discussed differences in the foundation assumptions of deviance theory by using a comparison of pre- and post-labeling perspectives. Gouldner and others (e.g., Liazos, 1972; Thio, 1973) used the concept of assumptions to demonstrate the presence of bias in sociology and, particularly, in work on deviance.

This interest in domain assumptions, world hypotheses, and paradigms has been instructive to theorists, especially those of a radical bent. Unfortunately, there is a tendency to impute a relatively immutable set of assumptions to theoretical positions and this immutability is questionable. The point many have ignored is that domain assumptions are also conceived from value sets and, therefore, can be imbued with outside characteristics. Thus, a theory does not have to be allied with singular assumptive frameworks but may over time have a succession of imputed backgrounds.

The question arises whether this is "bad" or not. Surely, the intent of the original theorist does not change, and one might argue that in that respect the original theory also does not change. On the other hand, a theory that does not provide insights and thereby change according to what is *seen* in it may not be as valuable as one that does. Maintaining only the original body of a theory does not serve integration very well either. Regardless, our Western culture heritage of thinking in a dualistic framework connotes a propensity to set up an either/or dichotomy: either *this* theory is correct or *that* theory is correct. Thus, reinterpreting theories tends to further the concept that theories are in competition.

COMPETING THEORIES

Theories are not just pronouncements about how crime and criminals happen, they are also a part of one's scholarly identity. It is this tendency that, combined with dualistic thought, helps set theories up as competing entities. The problem of competition has been singularly problematic. Adherents to individual theories often see themselves as having a grasp on "truth," in opposition to those who then appear to be somewhat "misguided" in their support of alternative positions.

Theoretical Interaction

In this regard Albert Cohen insightfully remarked in his work combining anomie and Chicago School traditions "it may be that we are confronted with a false dichotomy, that we are not really forced to choose between two conflicting theories. . . . If this is so, then the task of theory is to determine the ways in which the two kinds of factors mesh or interact" (1955:17). Cohen's comments suggest that different levels of theoretical analysis exist,[4] and a reasonable task is to find ways in which they can be made compatible. Indeed, the dualistic propensity to see "old" and "new" theories reduces the likelihood that compatibility issues will even be pursued. The old, through imputation of competing assumptions, cannot be part of the new. Some theorists, among them those who pursue theory integration, even go so far as to argue that using less than the entirety of a theory is unacceptable and that nothing must conflict (particularly imputed assumptions) when theories are integrated (see Hirschi [1979] for an argument against any form of integration and the essays in Messner, Krohn and Liska [1989] for the variety of views on the feasibility of theory integration).

Level of Explanation

In actuality, very few criminological theories find themselves in direct competition because they attempt to explain different parts of the crime/criminal dilemma. Some theories focus on crime and law, while others focus on criminal behavior or crime rates. Moreover, some criminologists have yet to become concerned with specifying the level of explanation (Short, 1985, 1989; Williams, 1981) of their favorite theory. Some theories attempt explanations at the level of structural relationships in society, while others attempt more processual explanations; some explain how large groups, or even societies, differ in their levels of crime while others attempt to explain individual level criminality. Finally, explanations vary by the age grouping of those whose behavior is being explained (e.g., "delinquency" versus "criminality" theories), or by whether the behaviors involve minor deviance or more serious forms of behavior. In truth, given this variety of explanation, few of our criminologically oriented theories compete directly with each other.

If this is so, then, what other reasons explain enthusiasm for theories among criminologists? I foresee two general explanations: (1) theories are found to be more or less supported by empirical evidence, and/or (2) criminologists are guilty of participating in fads and fashions in either theoretical or methodological orientation.

EMPIRICAL SUPPORT OR FASHION AND FAD?

What "evidence" can I offer that theories are as much products of ideology, values, and fad as they are based on the strength of empirical evidence? First, others have felt the same way. C. Wright Mills even uses the term "fad" in a discussion of "enthusiasms . . . [that] leave little or no intellectual trace" (1959:13). As already noted above, Alvin Gouldner (1970) argued that domain assumptions and world hypotheses were the very mainstay of theory and sociology in general. Similarly, Robert Bohm (1981) has argued forcefully that social theory and ideology are equivalent, and a large number of critical criminologists have taken the position as gospel. But there is another way to demonstrate this position: by taking a trip through modern criminological history.

Pre-Twentieth-Century Criminology

The beginnings of modern criminology are usually traced to the Classical School. That school was mainly a philosophical and political position regarding the nature of men and their relationship to the state. In short, it required no evidence for its position, although much of its humanism was indeed based on personal observations made by various authors. The following approach, the Positivist School, was much more evidence based. However, in truth, its emergence was a product of scientific evolution philosophy, the ascendance of industrialism and capitalism, and the rising status of medicine. The relatively new industrial system required values which both decried idleness and justified the new social order. A social Darwinism admirably emphasized both values by framing success in evolutionary terms. The field of medicine had been moving toward "scientific" status and seized the new field of criminal anthropology as an opportunity to demonstrate its ability to isolate physiological pathologies (Lindesmith and Levin, 1937: 669). As a result, it makes more sense to argue that the Positive School arose from values derived from the emergent social order rather than new evidence which it attempted to explain.

The Chicago School

American sociology produced the next identifiable "school" of thought with the work of the Chicago School. That school represented a break in values from the positivist pathological explanations of deviance. Their impetus came from a combination of popular reform movements, the emergence of sociology as a discipline, large-scale immigration and, finally, the beginnings of the Depression. Given this situation, Chicago criminologists could not locate pathology in the individual and, instead, found it in the social environment. Moving from geologically-linked social influences to social transmission of values, these scholars tended to view deviant people as situationally "normal" and crime as a function of situation and circumstance. Their theoretical approaches were derived from their sociological frame of reference and social events. Even though the Chicago School invented evidence methodologies, those methodologies supported their perspectives rather than created them.

The East Coast School

On the heels of the Chicago School, one might argue that the East Coast School represented by the work of Talcott Parsons and Robert Merton was indeed a product of methodology. The work of the Chicago School creating statistical methodology focused on rates of social phenomena was instrumental in contributing to the rise of a structural criminology. On the other hand, there is also substantial evidence that Merton was influenced by the newly translated work of Durkheim, the Depression, and emerging governmental emphasis on reform. Indeed, it appeared that social institutions were gaining popularity as "explanations" of societal events. Given the popular Depression-era belief that government was responsible for society's problems, Robert Merton's introduction to Emile Durkheim's work by Pitirim Sorokin provided a ready-made explanation for that belief: Society was simply in a state where the cultural goals and the societally approved means no longer worked together. Moreover, it appeared that this had become a permanent state for certain segments of society. Thus, methodology did not create the theoretical position, but it did work to support it. Subsequent theoretical positions (Cohen, Cloward, and Ohlin) were largely artifacts of a popular position that crime was tied to urban areas and delinquency to gangs, not new methodology nor evidence.

Labeling and Conflict Perspectives

The advent of labeling and conflict theories may be seen as a reaction of criminology to the new evidence of self-report studies. In this light, the new perspectives represent a departure from older theories which were based on official statistics. In one important epistemic way, then, method becomes theory and theory becomes method. This reciprocal connection appears time and time again in criminological theory. However, there is more than just a theory-research connection. An examination of the social context of the period shows an era of concern for civil rights, equality among men, and reaction to the authority of the state. To put it another way, the period was one of social protest and civil unrest. Labeling and conflict theories represent such similar concerns that one may reasonably assert that the new theories were as much a product of the values of the period as a response to new evidence failing to support older theories. Actually, radical theorists have never claimed to be tied to empirical evidence.

Social Control Theories

Social control theories have been seen as directly tied to self-report methodology, so there is some contention that these theories are indeed evidence based. However, social control theories existed prior to the self-report methodology. An examination of the social conditions suggests that the popularity of social control is more a product of a concurrently emerging conservatism concerned with the state of the family, education, religion, and national identity. These concerns are expressly reflected in contemporary social control theories (see Gottfredson and Hirschi [1990] for an argument that assigns primacy to early childhood socialization at the same time that parenting and single-parent families were of social concern). Again, it remains arguable whether self-report delinquency evidence accounts for the popularity of social control theories or merely serves to support a theoretical movement that matches social events of the time.

Contemporary Theories

Finally, the criminological theories of the 1980s were, in part, based on new victimological evidence. They were also based on disenchantment with explaining criminal behavior and a return to environmental concerns. Lifestyle and routine activities perspectives expressly focused on victim behavior and environmental conditions that increased the chances of a criminal event. Lawrence Cohen and Marcus Felson (1979) even went so far as to say that their concern with routine activities was purposely devoid of motivation theory. Rational theories were less based on a methodology than on the conservative mood of the times. Following the rise of deterrence and demise of rehabilitation, the public's approach to criminals was to give them what they "deserved" for their purposeful transgressions. Rational theories merely provided a rationale of reassurance that criminals were, indeed, purposeful. Both theories contain a strong element of moving toward the tenor of the times and a lesser element of following evidence. Certainly, there is little basis for inferring that the "new" theories were generated by new evidence.

Implications

So what may be concluded from this "history" of criminological schools? Perhaps the most basic conclusion is that criminology is generally affected by a sensitivity to social issues. Indeed, it would be even more surprising if that were *not* the case because criminology is predominantly a social science and crime itself is a social construction. Even more intuitive is the fact that criminology reflects emergent social issues and concerns. Importantly, though, the field often casts aside what came before without a reason other than the trendiness of the new position. And therein the danger lies: to set aside previous work is to set aside its insights as well. Moreover, such a propensity sets up theories from different schools as competing theories, even though they may not be.

PARADIGMS

While I believe a good case can be made for the fashions and fads argument, especially to explain the popularity of theories, criminological paradigms probably do exist. Some would argue that we have changed paradigms in the past: perhaps from the Chicago School to the East Coast School (structural functionalism) to labeling to social control to rational choice. While this may be true, it is more likely that these are not paradigms. Rather, these perspectives themselves are based on *how we know*.

Evidence Paradigms

The question of how we know is the same as asking what evidence is available to us and how we develop that evidence. I find the method of evidence production to be a much more compelling argument for paradigm status than the theories themselves. In addition, this is much closer to the way in which Kuhn viewed paradigms (the standardized use of exemplars). There are some rather clear evidence paradigms in criminology.

From Ethnography to Rates

In the first half of this century, two major forms of evidence paradigms were developed with entirely different implications for theory. The Chicago School theorists practiced field studies, or ethnography, and their knowledge came from observing people in different subcultures and groups where they lived and as they acted. True, the Chicago School also developed aggregate statistical methodologies, but those methodologies were used in a supplementary fashion to describe the areas in which people lived. The real use of statistical methodology was in the East Coast School. The structural functionalists had a much better purpose for statistical methodology: the construction of social abstracts. Thus, for them the epistemology was based on aggregate data, not studies of the individual nor even of small groups. Proper information came from rates and indices and that, in turn, required explaining through structural theories.

From Rates to Self-Reports

The labeling perspective of the 1960s turned on the ethnographic concerns of the Chicago School, indeed, it was derived from that school. However, a substantial part of the labeling perspective was a critique of the use of rates to establish reality. Rather than developing into a theoretical structure based on ethnography, a new methodology (self-report surveys) became dominant. The new task became to explain these results, which were somewhat divergent from rate-based knowledge. Thus, theories now were based on knowledge that suggested greater equality in offending among races and classes and required alternative variables. Social control theories became popular because they provided such variables.

From Self-Reports to Victimization Data

The final evidence paradigm was the development of the victimization survey. While ostensibly telling us something about offenders, the actual data told us about victims and the places they were victimized. Around this, our contemporary knowledge paradigm grew up, and theories were developed to explain time, place, and situation. Conversely, the de-emphasis on offenders resulted in theories that saw offenders in simpler terms: offenders were rational beings, making their own decisions, and were assumed to be less influenced by psychological and sociological variables. Now the primary task was to explain interaction between offender, victim, and environment. However, because victimization data is derived from survey methodology, the epistemology remains at the aggregate level just as it has since the final days of the Chicago School.

Combining Paradigms with Fashions and Fads

It is also true that none of the methodologies have actually *disappeared.* In each time of change, preceding methodologies remained and scholars continued to examine their evidence. What did occur, however, was that with the rise of the *new* methodology, the dominant amount of work became devoted to it and new theories were proposed to explain the findings of the new methodology. In short, the most interesting work and the more interesting questions were derived from the new evidence. And this is why I refer above to the effect of fashions and fads. True, I am now arguing that there have been paradigms in criminology—the paradigms of ethnography, rate-based statistics on offenders, self-report offender surveys and, finally, victimology surveys. It is the *evidence* epistemology that creates paradigmatic status, not the theories. And I think we are now possibly moving toward new evidence epistemology.

BASIC PROBLEMS OF THEORY

The preceding discussion focused on reasons for theories becoming popular (and sometimes dominant), or even being presented in the first place. The main goal was to achieve an appreciation that theory construction is intimately tied to outside factors and popularity is not merely a product of which theory has the greatest objective support. Having done that, I now wish to discuss the various elements that have prevented theories from directly reflecting reality. A common stance taken by criminological scholars is that the social world is immensely complex, with the ensuing implication that the theoretical enterprise is also immensely difficult. Therefore, we may assume that both the large number of theories and the value placed on them is a direct product of social complexity. However, there are reasons for our theoretical problems other than the mere complexity of reality.

Disciplinary Blindness

Since the 1920s, most criminological theories have been sociological in nature. Some, however, have been either biologically or psychologically based. Regardless of their particular orientation, a problem is evident: Criminological theories are disciplinarily reductionistic—they tend to focus on concepts derived from a single discipline. In fact, mainstream criminological theorists have been unabashedly enthusiastic in declaring the primacy of social factors in explaining criminal behavior and crime. One obvious reason for this state of affairs has been the dominance of criminology by scholars with sociology backgrounds. Scholars from other disciplines have been less prominent but, even so, have also been guilty of reifying their own chosen field of study. Regardless of the disciplinary content of the theories, they remain reductionistic as long as they contain concepts derived primarily from one discipline.

Clearly, human behavior is dynamic and interactive. That is, the behavioral system is a function of factors acting in concert to produce specific behaviors or patterns of behavior. I assume that, in concert with the general appearance of the universe, this system of factors is exceedingly complex and complicated. Moreover, these factors are derived from major dimensions. These dimensions, at the risk of oversimplification, can be referred to as biological, psychological, environmental, and social. Their components or factors are not necessarily isolated within each separate dimension; biological factors do not merely interact with and influence other biological factors but also interact with factors in other dimensions as well.

While the form of interaction *may* occur chiefly within specific dimensions, it will not necessarily occur in any particular instance. Further, the temporal order of factor interactions is not necessarily confined to the general temporal order of specific dimensions. For example, most biological factors are set in place at birth. However, it is also true that other biological influences may occur at various stages of life, and they may even be the most recent factors prior to the emission of a behavior. Jeffery (1977, 1989a), in reporting on biological research, even argues that there is a *continuing* interaction of the biological with the environmental.

These observations also imply that any interaction among various levels of factors is likely to be nonlinear. Depending on their order of introduction, the various disciplinary factors may even change their effect in nonlinear ways. Moreover, it is probable that simple recursive (one-way) models of causality are too simplistic in interactive systems. The feedback from change at various times can be logically expected to act on earlier components of the system.[5] Thus, nonrecursive models are probably more dependable ways of capturing reality.

I do not mean to suggest that criminology has been ignorant of disciplinary reductionism, although the recognition is indeed scant. As the most identifiable proponent, Ray Jeffery has eloquently argued for an interdisciplinary behavioral science (and criminology) for a number of years (1971, 1978, 1989b). I also do not mean to suggest here that existing theories are not dealing with complex ideas and concepts. Indeed, they do (see for instance, Vila, 1994) and for that reason alone they are more difficult to test. What I mean to convey is that they tend to focus on single-discipline variables and do so as they apply to specific points in time. This smacks of disciplinary hegemony — each discipline mostly attempts to explain behavior as if its "own" variables are the only ones that are really important. Surely, we have not been successful enough to justify that hubris.

Questionable Evidence

If one looks across the criminological discourse, a startling conclusion might be that there is not much to objectively demonstrate that any one theory is better than any other. I come to this conclusion based on reading the defenses of the various theories and the methodological critiques offered immediately following any substantial test of a theory, and my own survey of the explanatory power found for each test of theory in recent journals.

Versions of Reality

I have observed that many theories are defended on the basis of what appropriately represents reality. One way this occurs is to argue that tests were made in inappropriate situations or that inappropriate variables were used: in short, the tester failed to understand the theory. While this may be true, the frequency of the charge suggests that either we do not educate scholars well in theory[6] or that the theory itself is not adequately presented. The later problem is not an uncommon one, as theoretical concepts are often left undefined. If this is unintentional, then the theorist needs to refine the theory. If it is intentional, then the theorist has left an avenue for refuting negative tests by declaring the variables were not proper ones. One certainly hopes for the former. The other way a test's reality is represented as inappropriate is through level of explanation. For instance, defenders of Merton's anomie theory uniformly argued that the proper reality is an abstract one—that is, a structural view of the world. Any test involving individuals is simply not appropriate; therefore survey data may be only used in the aggregate to test a structural theory. Moreover, Mertonian theory views deviance as a great generality. Testing with dependent variables such as crime is being too specific—after all, the theory does not predict *which* mode of adaptation will be chosen, merely that the rates of various forms of deviance will be higher as the means/goals disjunction increases. Other theories have similarly constructed realities that allegedly require specific forms of tests (e.g., Hirschi and Gottfredson, 1993). Finally, I observe that even when a theory is supported by a test, opponents may argue these same points in an attempt to discredit the test. In short, they may suggest that its concepts were improperly measured.

Methodological and Statistical Error

Another form of defense is to critique (or otherwise dismiss) the methodology and statistical analysis of theoretical tests. While this is certainly well within the appropriate realm of scientific skepticism, a close examination of the commentary in the back of major journals yields a tit-for-tat form of critique and rebuttal (e.g., Chamlin and Cochran 1995, 1996; Jensen, 1996). In these commentaries the argument is often over the proper usage and interpretation of a statistical test, when the differential approaches are separated by a minuscule degree of error.[7] For instance, whether a factor analysis is accomplished by quartimax or equamax rotation[8] rarely changes the variables falling into the various factors and, even should that happen, the result affects only a variable or two. Tight bounds of error are important when theoretical models have been tightly elaborated and nuances become important. Such conditions are rarely the case. Similarly, sample parameters and sampling techniques are questioned; the type of data collection (secondary official records, surveys, self-reports) becomes an issue. In most of these discussions, there is no real estimation of the degree of error created by the alleged problems and the mere mention of error is sufficient to set the results aside. Such a position is, of course, untenable and in many cases simply another way to demonstrate bias for or against the theory.

Explanatory Power

It may also be that the level of empirical evidence used to support and refute almost all existing theories is questionable. Indeed, it appears to me that the various tests of theory are mostly lacking in any convincing level of explanatory power. By this I mean that the statistical tests, appropriate or not, generally tend to produce low correlations and explained variance. Theories most commonly pronounced as having the strongest levels of support in recent years include social control, social learning, and differential association (and integrated theories using these as main ingredients).Yet what constitutes "strong" levels of support is debatable. My impression of most published research results over the past twenty years is that somewhere between 5 percent and 25 percent of the variance in criminal/delinquent behavior or crime rates is commonly explained by individual theories.

Because this impression may not apply to recent research, I examined five years of theoretical tests published in *Criminology* and *Justice Quarterly*. Both are considered the most important journals of criminology and criminal justice and should, therefore, produce representative examples of good research. I found 18 studies, excluding deterrence research, with a total of 42 tests of theories (most tested more than one theory). While not all of these were decipherable in a "explained variation" fashion, those that were produced a range of 5 percent to 38 percent of the variance for the different theories.[9] Some of the tests reported only a multiple correlation that included a myriad of variables (controls, demographics, various theories, etc.); those tests purported to explain 12 percent to 64 percent of the variance. Because many of the studies used several variables to test even one theory, there were ranges of explained variance even within the studies. The average, across all theories and for all theoretical variables, was 13 percent explained variance for singular (one theory) results and 18 percent for aggregate (multiple correlation) results. In sum, it seems that my earlier impression of the average explanatory power of our theories still holds. On the whole, our efforts have not been entirely successful. For some theories, however, stronger evidence exists—particularly the differential-association/learning-theory version of delinquent peers and integrated theories, such as those proposed by Elliott *et al.* (1985).

Plausible Reasons for a Lack of Evidence

There are some general explanations for this state of affairs. One, the theories may not be very good. Two, the operationalization of the theoretical concepts may be generally inadequate, so we cannot demonstrate what exists. Three, our statistical methods may be inadequate to the task of demonstrating what exists. Perhaps the answer is all three, or a combination of them. In any of the three cases (or the three combinations), major work is necessary.

The first explanation is, in one sense, the essence of this chapter. Our theories are on the whole uni-dimensional, simplistic constructions of reality. Yet at the same time, I will argue that they do have complexity and do reflect reality, albeit a small portion of it. That "small portion" is the largest problem. A few theories, Reckless's containment theory[10] for example, are poorly constructed and somewhat illogical—but those are the exception. It is also true that many theorists have left their independent variables somewhat unspecified. This is part of the problem of operationalization (or conceptualization).

The second explanation is that we are not yet adequately translating the theoretical concepts into appropriately measured variables. This rationale, that of a paucity of operationalization, is treated in the next chapter under the material on conceptualization. Here, it will suffice to say that there are two sources of failure to properly conceptualize. First, there is the theorist's failure to fully explain the concepts and variables in the theory. Returning to Reckless's theory as an example, there is no clear explanation of the self-concept. Reckless says that the self-concept is not personality, yet it is internal. Moreover, external forces have virtually no effect when the self-concept is a bad one, yet he presents a 2 by 2 typology of the effects of inner and outer containment. The second source of failure is the researcher's inability to understand the theory and thereby properly measure the presumed independent variables. This failure is the fodder of much commentary in literature reviews and in comments and rebuttals in journals. Perhaps due in part to greater emphasis on methodological sophistication than on an understanding of theory, many researchers simply *approximate* theoretical concepts with variables that are handy in the secondary data they use.[11] While both sources assist in creating difficulties of testing theory, I believe there is ample evidence that researchers are more guilty than are the theorists.

The third explanation, inadequate statistical methodology, is also discussed in a following chapter. Here, I shall simply say that most of our statistical techniques assume linear relationships and normal distributions, while there is adequate evidence that reality is more complex than that. Moreover, the number of variables that can be used in some multivariate techniques is similarly limited, often by a requirement for some minimal number of cases per variable. Other restrictions exist for virtually all sophisticated statistics. Given this, there should be reasonable doubt that modeling complex behaviors, in complex environments, and with complex social relations is easily accomplished by current statistical tools. Though the statistical techniques exist by which to model such complexity, they are infrequently used in the social sciences.

In fairness, I do not mean to locate a lack of evidence in any particular one of these explanations. Indeed, the problem probably derives from a combination of all three (and other reasons as well). It is more likely that statistical problems, methodological problems, and ideological defenses all come into play to prevent most theories from having a fair test. In the face of this, though, one has to wonder how different groups can claim that *their* theory is "best" when most theories have a similar degree of supporting evidence. If one assumes that the level of support available to our current (and past) theories is relatively small, the clear implication is that we need to include "better" variables, perhaps arrayed in different logical patterns, and test them appropriately. Regardless, it seems that without strong empirical support, the popularity of any theory may be alternatively explained by ideological orientations.

Level of Abstraction

There are really three criminologies: a statistical, aggregate criminology, a social-psychological criminology, and an "in-between" criminology. The first works with criminological abstracts and concerns itself with rates of behavior. It is represented in structural theories explaining the effect of social institutions. This criminology is the dominant one today and largely has been since the 1950s. The second criminology is concerned with individual and small group behavior. It is represented largely in theories focusing on the process of becoming deviant. Found mostly among the Chicago School symbolic interactionist approaches, this criminology is rather dormant today. The third criminology serves as a bridge between the other two. Its task is to translate the findings of social-psychological criminologists into social abstracts understandable by the statistical criminologists (and vice versa). It is represented largely by theories of subculture and ecology, and, even though it is alive today, the relative dormancy of social-psychological criminology yields a dearth of translatable concepts. Its heyday was in the 1950s and 1960s, with attempts to merge Chicago School and East Coast School criminologies.

Our contemporary problem is that the most abstract version of criminology has become too dominant. This means that we tend to see crime and criminals not as an event or as persons but instead as problems of larger groups—even of social classes and societies—and it is those larger groups we are hell-bent on explaining. There is nothing inherently wrong in such a position; instead it is the *dominance* of the position that causes us to ignore events and people, to forget there is a process of deviance that must be investigated. This is, of course, encouraged by the corresponding dominance of statistical methodology over qualitative approaches. To continue to focus on statistical criminology is to continue to examine the shadows of interpersonal reality — something lingers and can almost be made out, yet its essence eludes us. On the other hand, qualitative criminology requires that one get involved and "dirty" one's hands in the research process (the degree of this may be appreciated by reading Jeff Ferrell's recent article in *Justice Quarterly* [1997]). All three levels of abstraction are necessary to an understanding of the crime experience.

Problems of Causality

A final explanation for at least some of our theoretical difficulties has to do with conceptions of causality. In most cases, cause is at best a background assumption for theories, rarely appearing as an explicit discussion.

Necessary Cause

While most of us would deny causal frameworks that include the concept of a necessary cause, there are still examples in criminological theory. Theories with this assumption focus on singular variables, such as an excess of definitions, and provide a deterministic view of the world. While this approach has some limited merit, it does belie substantial evidence that the social world is exceedingly complex. A bit more complex are theories that propose conditions that are necessary but not sufficient, such as status deprivation leading to delinquency. In this case, the effect changes to a probabilistic one where the introduction of the condition raises the probability of occurrence above zero, while the insufficiency condition keeps the probability below one. The single condition, however, suggests a relatively high probability.

Contingent Causality

More in alliance with the complexity issue are theories that suggest that a group of variables, taken together and contingent on each other, are sufficient to cause an effect.[12] Ecological and social-disorganization theory is an excellent example of this approach, where the identified elements such as vacant and condemned homes, "broken windows," and structural inequality serve as a contingent combination of sufficient variables. The causal problem here, from the standpoint of complexity, is that the "social disorganization" represents a singular construct and the contingent elements are merely different fragments of that concept. Thus, there is indeed recognition of complexity, yet only within one concept.

Probabilistic Causality

More recent probabilistic constructions of causality have many of the same problems. Under this approach a cause is assumed to be neither necessary nor sufficient but, instead, a "partial" cause (i.e., a variable that may partially influence another variable only some portion of the time). Potential causal variables are judged statistically, usually on the portion of explained variation they contribute to a mathematical model of the presumed relationship. Parsimony dictates that variables with the highest amount of explained variation be considered "causes," requiring that other variables with low amounts of variation be largely ignored. The operationalization issue looms even larger here. Insufficiently measured concepts, or concepts that share properties, can become more or less important in a model merely because of the variance in their measurement, not because of their theoretical validity. An allied issue is a tendency to deny causal status to any unobserved and unmeasured concept (this is not a direct problem for latent-structures analysis). Either all potential causal variables (and concepts) are included in the mathematical models or exogenous causality is denied. Certainly, we know that partitioning variance is problematic for causality when unmeasured variables exist, and we also know that criminologists are not yet omniscient. Thus, complexity can generate serious problems for probabilistic causality.

Proximate Causality

Proximate causality deals with the time-ordered relationship between variables. In effect, the general approach assumes that those independent variables closest in time (proximate variables) to the dependent variable are more likely to be "causes." While I realize that there is a long-standing recognition of what Paul Lazarsfeld (1955) called interpretation (intervening and mediating variables, or today's "indirect effects"), the tendency to look for variables close in time to the dependent variable still exists.

This is a problem in complex relationships where, in reality, the effect is either of long duration or spontaneous. Thus, a proximate-causality assumption may result in one of the following three threats to causality.

First, in a situation where many variables occur just prior to the presumed effect, it is possible to view any one as a probable effect, thus resulting in a search for the conditions under which one takes precedence over the others. The ensuing situation may produce inconsistent explanations, precipitating a choice of variables based on several different rationalizations and perhaps ultimately generating little of interest.

Second, closely temporal variables may be perceived as the cause based on preconceived notions of what those variables *should* be. Because theorists and researchers are unable to come to observations sans a priori knowledge, attributions of causality are threatened by continual misperceptions. If the closely temporal variables are regularly observed, then the threat to theory is magnified because the regularity itself can be taken to suggest validity of the causal attribution.

Third, observed proximate variables may be an artifact of methodological paradigms. In this case, certain variables are regularly included as mainstays of specific methodologies. For instance, official crime statistics contain only a few demographic variables, and these variables have been consistently used as important factors in theoretical formulations. Other evidence methodologies, such as self-report, have produced different theories. Moreover, these methodologies are generally not capable of producing evidence of temporal relationships, and, therefore, correlational magnitudes take priority with both time-order and proximity inferred as a product of the correlation itself.

CONCLUSIONS

I have tried to present a case in this chapter for the view that theory construction is relatively constrained. Some of this constraint has to do with the sensitivity of social scientists to the cultural events and changes of the day. Other explanations deal with an overweening emphasis on quantitative, statistical analysis and the strong tendency toward disciplinary reductionism.

How can these things have happened and, once they have happened, why is it that we do not simply say our farewells and move along? Two major reasons come to mind. First, we have maintained the primacy of the same general approaches for so long that we rarely question the way they reflect on reality. Indeed the extended primacy of the approaches means that we have built up a "scientific" language around them that, literally, *protects* them from questioning. Because language contains the symbols of thought, as we learn to think in a language it is those very linguistic conventions that shackle us. How do I come to this conclusion? Because I have frequently heard colleagues express the feeling that their data don't really seem to be accurate measures of what they are examining, but they continue to use them anyway. I have heard students express dismay that their experiences don't match our "objective" reality. And finally, I have sat in courtrooms, been in correctional facilities and police departments, and talked with "criminals" and I can assure you that the secondary data collected in those situations do not reflect the actual situations.

The second reason for continuing the status quo is literally that we have too much vested in the current epistemology. Our educational systems are as much to blame here as anything else we do. We train people to think and to perceive reality. For all our efforts to emphasize rationality, systematic thought, and critical reasoning, those things are not independent of reality. Education actually creates a pseudo-knowledge. We cannot know the truth but we can learn to *perceive* it differently. Indeed, we perceive it in such a fashion as it becomes useful to us. The burning question is "useful for what"? If the answer is allied to the mode of perception itself, then knowledge, truth, and reality become tautological.

Regardless of these problems, there are currently some promising "new" approaches to examine. Lifespan and change theories are at least questioning the rather static nature of our criminological view. Postmodernist theories are questioning everything from linguistic metaphors in law to the conflict approach endemic in the way we treat and work with people (peacemaking). Whether these "new" perspectives are correct or not, some value still remains in forcing consideration of alternative perspectives for examining human behavior and social constructions.

NOTES

1. I would like to thank Gil Geis for suggesting this latter reason.

2. Some of what follows is adapted from comments in "The Sociology of Criminological Theory: Paradigm or Fad" (Williams, 1981).

3. Scholars are still arguing over the values and assumptions behind differential association (see Kornhauser, 1978; Hirschi and Gottfredson, 1979; Matsueda, 1988; Akers, 1996; Hirschi, 1996) and anomie theory (Hirschi, 1969; Cohen, 1993; Bernard, 1987; McShane and Williams, 1985). Other discussions have developed around the assumptions of virtually every popular theory.

4. Methodologists refer to this as a "unit of analysis" problem.

5. See John Hagan (1993) for an example of the reciprocal effects of unemployment and crime at the individual level. He documents that unemployment is so embedded in the social structure that it affects an individual's motivation toward crime and subsequently that crime affects an individual's opportunities for employment. Thus, a cycle is born (something that labeling theory also tells us). Additionally, Terence Thornberry (1987), in his interactional theory of delinquency, argues that causal factors are reciprocal over the life course, with delinquency being the effect and the cause of weakened social control.

6. This is a problem in graduate education that has already been treated in the first chapter.

7. Also see the commentary concerning error in Chapter 5.

8. This is an arbitrary choice of statistical techniques although it was the bone of contention in series of anomie studies by Lander (1954), Bordua (1958–59), and Chilton (1964). For the same statistic, I could make a similar argument for the extraction technique (for instance, rarely is there any substantial empirical difference between principal-components, maximum-likelihood or alpha-factor extractions). For other statistics, such as discriminant analysis, whether one uses Rao's V or Wilkes' lambda to identify the degree of separation between the functions is normally of little import to error.

9. It appears that the modern style of statistical analysis is to report multiple correlations for an entire model and effect sizes for the individual

variables. The commentary then surrounds those variables with significant effect sizes. Because the effects (at least in varieties of multiple regression) are usually slope estimates (standardized or not), it becomes impossible to determine how much of the total variance they contribute. A large effect size may be barely significant and virtually negligible in its contribution to the total variance.

10. Walter Reckless'(1961: 335–359) theory of containment, or self-concept, is a particularly good example of the failure to properly and logically construct a theory. A story related to me by Frank Scarpitti (who was one of Reckless' students) will help to explain. When Sutherland died, Reckless assumed that the mantle of dean of American criminology had fallen on him. There was one major problem: the dean of criminology was supposed to have a theory of criminal behavior and Reckless had proposed none. Thus, he scrambled to construct a new theory, different from others in existence. The resulting theory was not well thought out and contained several contradictions (not to mention that his research to prove the theory might be seen as better evidence for labeling).

11. Virtually *any time* secondary data are used in theory testing there is a great likelihood that the variables used to represent a theory do not do so adequately. By definition, the variables were used because they were handy, not because they were the best representations.

12. There is also, of course, the essentialist position that a group of variables necessarily and sufficiently predicates a cause. I do not ascribe that extremist position to any criminological theorist, although some may wish to make such a case.

REFERENCES

Akers, Ronald L. (1996). Is differential association/social learning cultural deviance theory? *Criminology* 34: 229–247.

Bernard, Thomas (1987). Testing structural strain theories. *Journal of Research in Crime and Delinquency* 24: 262–280.

Bohm, Robert M. (1981). Reflexivity and critical criminology. Pp. 20–47 in Gary F. Jensen (ed.) *Sociology of Delinquency: Current Issues.* Beverly Hills, CA: Sage.

Bordua, David J. (1958–59). Juvenile delinquency and "anomie": An attempt at replication. *Social Problems* 6: 230–238.

Chamlin, Mitchell B., and John K. Cochran (1995). Assessing Messner and Rosenfeld's institutional anomie theory: A partial test. *Criminology* 33: 411–429.

Chamlin, Mitchell B., and John K. Cochran (1996). Reply to Jensen. *Criminology* 34: 133–134.

Chilton, Roland J. (1964). Delinquency area research: Baltimore, Detroit, and Indianapolis. *American Sociological Review* 29: 71–83.

Cohen, Albert K. (1955). *Delinquent Boys: The Culture of the Gang*. New York, NY: Free Press.

Cohen, Albert K. (1993). Letter to the author. January 29.

Cohen, Lawrence E., and Marcus Felson (1979). Social change and crime rate trends: A routine activities approach. *American Sociological Review* 44: 588–607.

Elliott, Delbert S., David Huizinga, and Suzanne S. Ageton (1985). *Explaining Delinquency and Drug Use*. Beverly Hills, CA: Sage.

Ferrell, Jeff (1997). Criminological verstehen: Inside the immediacy of crime. *Justice Quarterly* 14: 3–23.

Gibbons, Don C. (1994). *Talking about Crime and Criminals: Problems and Issues in Theory Development in Criminology*. Englewood Cliffs, NJ: Prentice Hall.

Gibbs, Jack P. (1966). Conceptions of deviant behavior: The old and the new. *Pacific Sociological Review* 9: 9–14.

Gibbs, Jack P. (1972). *Sociological Theory Construction*. Hinsdale, IL: Dryden.

Goffman, Erving (1959). *The Presentation of Self in Everyday Life*. Garden City, NY: Doubleday Anchor Books.

Gottfredson, Michael, and Travis Hirschi (1990). *A General Theory of Crime*. Stanford, CA: Stanford University Press.

Gouldner, Alvin, W. (1970). *The Coming Crisis of Western Sociology*. New York, NY: Basic Books.

Hagan, John (1993). The social embeddedness of crime and unemployment. *Criminology* 31: 465–491.

Hamm, Mark (1996). Review of *Incapacitation: Penal Confinement and the Restraint of Crime* (Zimring and Hawkins). *Justice Quarterly* 13: 525–530.

Hirschi, Travis (1979). Separate and unequal is better. *Journal of Research in Crime and Delinquency* 16: 34–38.

Hirschi, Travis (1969). *Causes of Delinquency*. Berkeley, CA: University of California Press.

Hirschi, Travis (1996). Theory without ideas: Reply to Akers. *Criminology* 34: 249–256.

Hirschi, Travis, and Michael Gottfredson (1979). Introduction: The Sutherland tradition in criminology. Pp. 7–19 in Travis Hirschi and Michael

Gottfredson (eds.) *Understanding Crime: Current Theory and Research.* Beverly Hills, CA: Sage.

Hirschi, Travis, and Michael Gottfredson (1993). Commentary: Testing the general theory of crime. *Journal of Research in Crime and Delinquency* 30: 47–54

Jeffery, C. Ray (1971). *Crime Prevention Through Environmental Design.* Beverly Hills, CA: Sage.

Jeffery, C. Ray (1977). *Crime Prevention Through Environmental Design,* 2nd ed. Beverly Hills, CA: Sage.

Jeffery, C. Ray (1978). Criminology as an interdisciplinary behavioral science. *Criminology* 16: 149–169.

Jeffery, C. Ray (1989a). *Criminology: An Interdisciplinary Approach.* Englewood Cliffs, NJ: Prentice Hall

Jeffery, C. Ray (1989b). An interdisciplinary theory of criminal behavior. Pp. 69–87 in William S. Laufer and Freda Adler (eds.) *Advances in Criminological Theory,* vol. 1. New Brunswick, NJ: Transaction.

Jensen, Gary (1996). Comment on Chamlin and Cochran. *Criminology* 34: 129–131.

Kornhauser, Ruth R. (1978). *Social Sources of Delinquency.* Chicago, IL: University of Chicago Press.

Lander, Bernard (1954). *Toward an Understanding of Juvenile Delinquency.* New York, NY: Columbia University Press.

Lazarsfeld, Paul F. (1955). Interpretation of statistical relations as a research operation. Pp. 115–125 in Paul F. Lazarsfeld and Morris Rosenberg (eds.) *The Language of Social Research.* New York, NY: Free Press.

Liazos, Alexander (1972). The poverty of the sociology of deviance: Nuts, sluts, and perverts. *Social Problems* 20: 103–120.

Lindesmith, Alfred, and Yale Levin (1937). The Lombrosian myth in criminology. *American Journal of Sociology* 42: 653–671.

Matsueda, Ross (1988). The current state of differential association theory. *Crime and Delinquency* 34: 277–306.

McShane, Marilyn D., and Frank P. Williams III (1985). Anomie theory and marijuana use: Clarifying the issues. *Journal of Crime and Justice* 8: 21–40.

Messner, Steven F., Marvin D. Krohn, and Allen E. Liska (eds.) (1989). *Theoretical Integration in the Study of Deviance and Crime: Problems and Prospects.* Albany, NY: State University of New York Press.

Mills, C. Wright (1959). *The Sociological Imagination.* New York, NY: Oxford University Press.

Reckless, Walter C. (1961). *The Crime Problem.* 3rd ed. New York, NY: Appleton-Century-Crofts.

Short, James F., Jr. (1985). The level of explanation problem in criminology. Pp. 51–72 in Robert F. Meier (ed.) *Theoretical Methods in Criminology.* Beverly Hills, CA: Sage.

Short, James F., Jr. (1989). Exploring integration of theoretical levels of explanation: Notes on gang delinquency. Pp. 243–259 in Steven F. Messner, Marvin D. Krohn, and Allen E. Liska (eds.) *Theoretical Integration in the Study of Deviance and Crime: Problems and Prospects.* Albany, NY: State University of New York Press.

Thio, Alex (1973). Class bias in the sociology of deviance. *American Sociologist* 8: 1–12.

Thornberry, Terence P. (1987). Toward an interactional theory of delinquency. *Criminology* 25: 863–891.

Vila, Bryan (1994). A general paradigm for understanding criminal behavior: Extending evolutionary ecological theory. *Criminology* 32: 311–359.

Wellford, Charles F. (1989). Towards an integrated theory of criminal behavior. Pp. 119–128 in Steven F. Messner, Marvin D. Krohn, and Allen E. Liska (eds.) *Theoretical Integration in the Study of Deviance and Crime: Problems and Prospects.* Albany, NY: State University of New York Press.

Williams, Frank P., III (1981). The sociology of criminological theory: Paradigm or fad. Pp. 7–19 in Gary F. Jensen (ed.) *Sociology of Delinquency: Current Issues.* Beverly Hills, CA: Sage.

Williams, Frank P., III (1984). The demise of the criminological imagination: A critique of recent criminology. *Justice Quarterly* 1: 91–106.

CHAPTER 4
Conceptualizing and Measuring

Just as there are dominant approaches to theory, so, too, are there dominant perspectives on how to conceive and measure reality. This chapter examines and critiques methods of conceptualization in much the same way the third chapter inquired into theory. The materials that follow inspect the contemporary method of perceiving reality and translating that perception into measurement. In general, I will argue that research emphases have swung so far toward technique that substance has been largely ignored. Technical detail and issues seem to have become more important than what we actually measure.

THE USE OF CONCEPTS[1]

Although I have already discussed some of the generic problems inherent in conceptualization and the use of concepts, some specific problems are important to criminology and criminal justice. This section explores problems in our dependent variable, crime, and the critical variables used to explain crime. I begin with the problem of classification.

Classification Schemes

If the social sciences are, indeed, to emulate the natural sciences, then one might expect the equivalent of a classification scheme as is in biological phyla. That is, there ought to be a scheme that classifies all social phenomena or, at the least, a sociological scheme that classifies humans. Given the importance of some sociological variables, one might be persuaded to say that it does exist. For instance, social class is clearly one of the most critical variables in sociology (if not *the* most critical variable) and is used to classify experiences, propensities, and expectations of people in a culture. On the other hand both race and gender seem to have equal claim as a classifying variable. Further, class, race, and gender overlap in their effect on people. In other words, all three variables interact to produce varied effects. Thus, there is no clear evidence that *any* proper typology exists for sociological study. Of course, there may be no good reason, other than emulation of the natural sciences, for such a classification scheme in the social sciences. A more pertinent question might be whether it would benefit the work of studying humans—and the answer to that question is not at all clear. But for those who would emulate the natural sciences, the question is a pressing one.

Definitions of Crime

In an ironic twist, one of the chief problems of criminology has always been its subject matter, i.e., how to classify illegal and deviant behavior. Crime, as is often stated, is a rather vague concept (Barak, 1995).[2] Leslie Wilkins (1968:477) even views definitions of crime as largely tautological. The various approaches to defining crime have ranged from generalized deviance (labeling theorists), through violations of human rights (conflict theorists; see especially, Schwendinger and Schwendinger, 1970), to acts registered in the criminal codes (consensus theorists; see especially, Tappan, 1947:100). All of these (and several other attempts at clarification) have served to further our understanding of the difficulties involved; none, however, are useful measures of criminality and criminal behavior (see Ball and Curry, 1995, for a recent acknowledgment of the problem and an attempt to rectify the definition problem in the study of gangs). Rather than working further on this critical problem, most criminologists acknowledge the various critiques, shake their heads knowingly, and proceed to use legal definitions of behavior (Sampson and Laub, 1993:252; Gottfredson and Hirschi, 1990:256).

This practice of tipping one's hat and proceeding as if legal crime were essentially synonymous with behavioral events is one of the contradictions of criminology. Criminologists know such an approach means that a political definition of crime is being used. And they know further that behaviors with identical action and intent, such as homicide and wartime heroism, are simultaneously abhorred and praised, depending upon the political interest behind the act. Thus, identical behaviors are both criminal and conforming under a legal definition of crime. Further, there are people who commit a criminal act who, because either they or the act are not discovered, are indistinguishable from those who are not criminals. The alternative, to use a self-report questionnaire that asks "have you ever. . . ," relates to the "dark figure" of crime but fails to clarify crime itself. The end product of most of our endeavors has been a critical dependent variable that has been reduced to the level of a questionable and unreliable construct.

Before proceeding to examination of legal definitions of crime, it would be wise to issue a quick disclaimer to those who think that, by the discussion above, I am uncritically advocating the use of a generalized, "deviance" version of crime. Such is not the case. The commonality of most generalized deviance (taking of small items, striking another, threatening another, etc.) makes it unlikely that these behaviors can be profitably used to describe crime.

The Effect of a Legal Definition of Crime

Why should this state of affairs remain? I believe that the answer is largely ideological. That is, there are cultural, political, and disciplinary belief systems at work among criminologists as in all disciplines. When these systems affect the central disciplinary concept, however, a dangerous situation develops. A rationalization that allows the legal definition of crime to be used as "the best alternative" is not merely an academically informed opinion brought about by objective consideration. It is also an ideological decision with unquestioned and implicitly buried definitions of behavior.

Such a rationalization, in fact, has three unfortunate byproducts. First, it produces disciplinary confusion. From a behavioral standpoint, crime and noncrime become conceptually overlapping categories with a subsequent increase in error variance. There are people who commit crimes who are not caught and people who do not commit crimes but are perceived to have done so (see Howard Becker's typology and discussion of the issue [1963:20]). The implications of this are that "criminal" and "noncriminal" are not mutually exclusive categories— and this is the minimal requirement for accurate measurement. Depending on the distribution of incorrectly classified cases, the dependent variable (crime) may be virtually useless. Self-report studies have shown that there is a healthy proportion of undiscovered criminality among the "noncriminal" public. Other than producing a poorly categorized dependent variable, the amount of potential error has ramifications for statistical analysis. Because most of the explained variance being produced by independent variables in current analyses is rather small, one may have problems determining if the explained variance is a product of error in the dependent variable or "real." In short, otherwise well-constructed, scientific investigation can easily be fraught with error rates larger than the expected effect of many independent variables.

I believe that an argument can be made for a multifaceted explanation of "criminality": thus, it may be entirely unreasonable to expect too much of any particular independent variable or even sets of independent variables, but this is another problem entirely. Situations in which crime and non-crime categories overlap require rather gross and general-purpose explanations in order to attribute systematic variance to some presumed cause. Under these conditions, it is difficult to construct explanations of criminality that will hold up to empirical test.

Second, the potential for creating a jaded and politically sensitive criminology is great. Continued failures to empirically validate theory will result in a pragmatic field which is critical of theory as, indeed, has been the case (see Wilson, 1982; Wilson and Herrnstein, 1985). Criminologists are certainly not going to forsake their *raison d'être*; they will simply adjust their focus toward more "productive" materials, such as police efficiency or community-oriented policing. Further, a pragmatic orientation is best focused on the criminal justice system itself, an area where the legal definition of crime is appropriate. This "new" focus actually denotes a shift in the subject matter of the field from criminal behavior to that of processing systems for criminals. Once behavior is no longer at issue, criminological resources will become devoted to furthering the aims of the criminal justice system.

The inherent political nature of the legal system forms a relatively dynamic and changing milieu of criminological issues. The choice of issues for inquiry is susceptible to political winds and, of course, funds being offered by various government agencies (e.g., National Institute of Justice, Office of Juvenile Justice and Delinquency Prevention, Bureau of Justice Statistics, Bureau of Justice Assistance, National Science Foundation) and private foundations (e.g., McArthur Foundation, Ford Foundation, Rockefeller Foundation). The end result, then, of an unquestioned acceptance of legal crime is that political images can come to be seen as proper guidance for scientific investigations, regardless of their ideological biases.

Third, the range of crime is greatly restricted by legal definitions. Any governmental structure has two main reasons for criminal legislation: public protection and self-interest. The latter is most clearly exemplified by those actions that are *not* defined as criminal. These are those behaviors arbitrarily defined as being in the governmental interest. Thus, a capitalistic society may allow certain banking practices (albeit regulated), a socialistic society may restrict human rights, and others may tacitly encourage traffic in illegal drugs. Not only does a legal definition of crime create problems in the differentiation of behavior within a society, but trans-societal analyses are rendered almost impossible. Terrorism, international drug dealing, arms trading, and environmental pollution are among a group of behaviors that, because of their very politicality, are difficult for most criminologists to claim as part of their domain.

One of the inherent problems, exemplified by the old debate between Paul Tappan (1947) and Edwin Sutherland (1945), is that officially crime is only behavior in violation of the criminal law. In this sense, criminology itself is a derivative of law: the name reflects a concern with crime. To argue that criminology may need to expand beyond crime is to play with the semantically ludicrous. That, perhaps, is the greatest problem: criminology is semantically bounded. To study analogous behavior (i.e., harmful and deleterious behavior) may require a new name for the discipline, else we engage in illogic. This is exemplified in critiques of Michael Gottfredson and Travis Hirschi's (1990:15) recent attempt to redefine crime in a more useful fashion as "acts of force or fraud undertaken in the pursuit of self-interest."

Some Reasons for Definitionally Related Problems

I believe there are some particular reasons that criminology finds itself in this state of affairs. Ironically, one of them is the very search for causes of criminal behavior itself. The intriguing search for these causes overshadows the mundane problem of defining crime. In addition, the very task of determining what we mean by criminal behavior may even require that causal explorations be temporarily set aside. Second, an even more mundane issue is that of adequate measurement, something with which the field has never had any burning desire to spend much time.[3] A closer examination of crime leads invariably to the necessity of establishing the reliability and validity of proposed measurement forms, a procedure long disdained in practice by many social scientists. Yet, there has not been, and probably will not be, funding or publication opportunities for such work.

Perhaps as important as any other force is the effect of the information age on criminology. The ability to produce, store, and access large datasets on computers has clearly changed the face of the discipline. Unfortunately, while the availability of these data encourages exploration of aggregate and structural variables, it also discourages the questioning of dependent variables. Closely tied to this profound new force is a practical consideration. The collection of bigger and better datasets is prohibitively expensive; so much so, that government agencies are the primary funding sources for such research. Because these agencies have their own agendas and internal considerations, the kinds of data being collected are directly connected to political interests and definitions of deviance. As the datasets are used to answer broader research questions, their effect grows.

Finally, and in conjunction with most of the forces above, the development of criminal justice as a discipline to study and assist the criminal justice system has been critical to the evolution of criminology. From the time of the 1967 President's Commission, criminal justice has been more interested in system efficiency and operation. Over the past dozen years, however, an increasing focus on moral responsibility and punitiveness intensified political interest in the efficiency of the criminal justice system. Scholars who espoused concern with etiological issues were increasingly at a disadvantage in the chase for research funds.[4] Many criminologists have resolved this dilemma by moving into criminal justice programs and/or taking up system-oriented issues. The other option, of course, has been to forsake original research and use the government databases noted above. Mainstream criminological interest in nonlegal, behavioral definitions of crime has consequently suffered.[5]

THE CONCEPTUALIZATION OF CRITICAL
EXPLANATORY VARIABLES

While there are many "critical" variables to the study and explanation of crime and delinquency, four of the most common are gender, race, age, and social class. Indeed, all four consistently have been found to be associated with criminality and crime rates. Years of careful investigation have produced a wealth of information; yet, at the same time and with the exception of social class, the field has not moved beyond a rudimentary conception of these variables. When compared to the meticulous identification and operationalization of more esoteric variables (e.g., cynicism), the sheer simplicity with which basic independent variables have been approached is astounding. In short, criminology has taken a rather rich set of concepts and reduced them to a measurement scheme which fails to capture even the essence of what we began with. In taking this stance, I am forced to state a heresy in order to make an explanation: Gender, race, age, and social class themselves have little to do with crime. That which they *represent*, however, is critical to an understanding of crime.

The Verstehen of Social Constructs

These variables, and others, are not in themselves characteristics of individuals that interest us. To make the point more directly, sex is merely a biological distinction. Age is merely a product of calendar time negotiated since birth. When we discuss these variables we imply much more, a *verstehen* of our cultural roles and ideologies; otherwise we would be delving into the realms of biochemistry and neurology. This *verstehen* is clearly the intent behind our use of the terms, yet the way we collect data and summarize their meaning belies this intent. In simpler terms, I am saying that these "simple" characteristics of people are, in reality, not that. They are instead very complex cultural constructions by which we express our beliefs, biases, and stereotypical imputations of group characteristics. Attempts to operationalize these constructions as simple variables and then treat them as if the constructs had been measured are not merely difficult, they require a different perspective. Such an approach is precisely the point behind recent research and thinking that rejects the biological term "sex" for a culturally informed "gender."

Complexity of the Variables

What, then, are these variables? How do they convey a richness of information that is not in our data? The answer to these questions lies in their use as surrogates for other, more complex variables that represent critical sociological relationships with criminality. While "sex" is a biological variable connoting the presence or absence of a Y chromosome, it has most commonly been used in the social sciences as a sociological composite of the roles and statuses of Western culture. It conveys relative economic and social power in defined situations as well as a profusion of other imputed information upon which others act and react. To be male does not mean simply that one has a Y chromosome but that a style of dress is worn, a certain posture is taken while speaking, or that one has a particular orientation toward life in general. In the words of Everett Hughes (1945) and Howard Becker (1963), sex[6] is a "master status" that results in the imputation of other attributes to an individual. Race, age, and social class are similarly rich in their conveyance of status and expectation.

Variables of this type then represent a shorthand way of cataloging the effects of culture, social roles, statuses, situations, and myriad other social expectations and events. When criminologists discuss the "effect of race on crime rates," they refer to the broader constellation of social reality, not the mere biological fact. This is a practice that results in the assignment of causal statements to variables that *have not been measured*. Clearly, such attributions are metaphysical by nature. As clarification, I do not object here to the use of correlations between, say, age and crime. However, age is not a causal (or an explanatory) factor; one must be able to say *why* age correlates with crime. This is currently a guessing game because we usually fail to provide the intuited concepts in our research.

It is one thing for a field to begin the measurement of critical variables in a rudimentary fashion; it is entirely another for that field to maintain the same level of measurement some fifty years later. Criminology needs to determine what is meant by the shorthand of race, gender, and age and find ways to measure those concepts. Only then will we determine the existence of critical social relationships we now only *assume* to exist.

Operationalizing Critical Social Concepts

While improved measurement of the concepts behind race, gender, age, and social class will be difficult, it should take place on two levels. First, the concepts involved have to be made overt and, second, various scales and measures need to be proposed and tested. I will briefly illustrate the first task here and leave the latter to specialists in the area of methodology, although it certainly would not be too difficult to include some simple measures on survey instruments to test their effect. Further, I will focus on social class, race, and age since gender theorists are already doing the important work of defining attributes of male and female roles in Western society (see Smart [1995] and Simpson [1991] for commentaries related to criminology and Lorber [1996] for an excellent discussion of the dichotomies inherent in the concepts of sex, sexuality, and gender), and social class is similarly being given attention. I also presume that those who specialize in social class, race relations, or youth or aging will have better ideas on the "meaning" of these three variables.

Social Class

Social class is virtually endemic to criminological theory either explicitly or implicitly. Social class began as a sociological construct measured by triangulated variables. That is, social class was originally conceived as an abstract station in life that could be used to describe the common experiences of large groups of people. In order to determine which social class one belonged to, a series of items was measured and assumed to present a composite picture of one's life station. For instance, researchers in the 1930s suggested characterizing social class in terms of such things as neighborhood, value of house, types of magazines subscribed to, use of language, and style of dress (e.g., Lynd and Lynd, 1937). In a rather strange turn of events, social class today tends to be characterized by a single variable or two, usually income and/or education. That these variables only partly reflect social class is not surprising. The question is why the practice continues. Surely an attorney's counsel to a client to appear in court wearing a suit, with a new haircut, and exhibiting "proper" demeanor is nothing more than an attempt to convey social class. In fact, the attorney seems to have a better notion of conveying social class than most social science researchers do when constructing variables for data collection. Fortunately, there is a movement to bring the missing range of variables back to measurements of social class.

Race

Perhaps the most obvious beginning for an understanding of racial roles and attributes is an examination of stereotypes. It should be clear that the essence of race has little to do with skin color or physical features. Instead, it focuses on attributes that are commonly associated with members of a race. Conflict theorists have long suggested that power is one of these characterizing attributes, be it economic or political. In the same vein, similarities and dissimilarities with the dominant culture assist in forming a view of race. These constitute such factors as style of dress, use of language (especially argot), and preferences in foods, music, and art. Demeanor and style of behavior are also implicated, although for criminology these aspects begin to tread directly on the issue of crime and deviance. In short, a good beginning for a determination of racially linked attributes is to ask what expectations we have of people.[7]

Another way to suggest the meaning of "race" is to examine it phenomenologically. Such an approach would concentrate on the subtle behaviors, gestures, and communications that provide information on individuals in various situations. A suitable, and telling, example for criminology is to compare a secondary data notation for race in the records of a criminal trial to the actual perceptions of members of the jury, the judge, and the prosecutor when "viewing" the defendant. True, this raises the problem of relativity in perception, but is this not closer to reality than a simple categorization of "white" or "black?" Such an example also points to possibilities of interaction among attributes.

Age

The attributes of age are in some ways similar to those of race. Certainly, previous literature has noted the powerlessness of youth and the disadvantaged economic position of many of the elderly. Stereotypically, American youth have been characterized by imputations of irresponsibility and impulsivity. I even have doubts that "delinquency," in its minor forms, is actually independent of these attributes. Rather than characterize the average criminal as "young," it may make more sense to determine what is meant by the term "young" and then look to see if levels of those variables among the population serve to explain deviance.

Moreover, whatever it is that we mean by "maturity" is important since certain stages in life are assumed to have different levels of maturity, demeanor, and preferences. It would be difficult, for example, to imagine many teenagers who prefer classical music and literature, French cuisine, and Renaissance art. In fact, to characterize that person as "sixteen years old" (as would be the case under typical measurements of age) would create serious problems of misinter-pretation. These attributes are associated with later stages in life as well as with particular segments of the population (an interaction with socioeconomic status). Concepts such as these are all worth exploring.

SIMPLICITY AS A FORCE BEHIND IMPROPER CONCEPTUALIZATION

The problem of measuring aggregate abstractions with single variables such as those above is not merely an issue of convenience. There are several precipitating factors behind their use, including scientific assumptions, measurement ideologies, and the difficulty of measuring composite abstractions. Each of these has a particular effect on social science research. It should be clear that measurement theory itself is critical to the way we observe and what we declare to be worth observing. Just as we produce theories of delinquent behavior, there is a set of assumptions about the way those theories are related to the world of observation. These assumptions, constituting an empirical theory of measurement, are part and parcel of the way science is pursued. While they are sometimes explicit, assumptions are most often implicit (see Selltiz, Wrightsman and Cook, 1976:38–42, for a more comprehensive coverage of the issues). Here, I simply want to raise the issues and make them obvious.

Parsimony

The first reason I can find for conceptual simplicity is simplicity itself. The philosophical assumptions behind science yield a belief that parsimony is desirable. This means that researchers are encouraged to reduce the number of variables in their research designs to a very few "important ones."[8] This tenet is derived from a truism that it is indeed difficult to interpret the complex relationships among a large number of variables. Therefore, in the interests of interpretability, one should use only those variables that capture the largest amount of variance in the dependent variable. Unfortunately, the search for parsimonious variables can lead one to forget that such variables often represent composites that are derived from several concepts. Or stated otherwise, these variables may merely be relatively meager proxies for other, more complex social, psychological, and biological dimensions.

Measurement Procedures

Ironically, the very issue of better measurement is also confounded by measurement procedures. Most social scientists have taken the approach that scientific objectivity is at its best when data observations are expressed in a quantitative fashion. While I have already treated this subject, it is still necessary to point out that measurement must adequately represent the phenomenon being quantified. Failure to do so results in numbers without meaning or, at the least, numbers that do not mean what the researcher pretends they do. I would contend that this problem is common.

Related to this problem, I believe, is the present dominance of a theory of measurement commonly called "levels of measurement." In 1946, S.S. Stevens published a paper in which he argued that the use of statistical techniques could be standardized by a recognition of the form of numerical information each required. The typology of numerical information he presented (nominal, ordinal, interval, and ratio) is now standard fare for any student taking a statistics or research methods course. What many do not know, however, is that Stevens based his theory of scales of measurement on the concept of invariance, that is, under what conditions might a mathematical group structure (general equation) retain its properties?

Logically beginning with the level he named "ratio," Stevens used the similarity group ($\chi' = \alpha\chi$) to define invariance only by multiplication by a constant. In this case, the numerals change in size, but not in relation to each other or the absolute zero point. He defined invariance in the "interval" class as the general linear group ($\chi' = \alpha\chi + b$), where the addition of a constant keeps the numerals in equidistant positions but results in an arbitrary zero. At the "ordinal" level, invariance is the isotonic group [$\chi' = f(\chi)$; where $f(\chi)$ means any monotonic increasing function] with multiplication by any increasing function. At this level, the concept of true distance is lost, and the numerals maintain invariance in their ordered positions. Finally, Stevens called the most unrestricted group of numerals the "nominal" class. Invariance here is the permutation group [$\chi' = f(\chi)$; where $f(\chi)$ means any one-to-one substitution]. These numerals are nothing more than labels and are equivalent to letters. Regardless of the result, the point is that Stevens used special cases of invariance to create his theoretical classes of numerals. Moreover, he tells us that the scheme "is not meant to imply that all scales belonging to the same mathematical group are equally precise or accurate or useful or 'fundamental'" (1946: 680). In short, there are mathematical operations and conceptual groupings to which his theoretical scale does not apply. The purpose of any measurement scale is merely to establish a consistent set of rules by which to interpret data.

How, then, is this important? Under this typology many assume that if a particular variable is measured as "nominal" then the concept it represents must also be nominal. This, of course, is not true; it may simply mean that the concept has been poorly operationalized. Thus, such variables as gender and race, while nominal in their usual measurement form, are in reality complex sociological concepts. The problem is that of poor conceptualization, precipitated by the fact that they have "always" been measured at a nominal level.

One of the reasons, and perhaps a primary one, for a general lack of ability to explain our dependent variables is that variance is lost when information otherwise available in our independent variables is destroyed by treating them as mere categories. Such measurements result from poor conceptualization, such as measuring age as "young," "middle-aged," and "elderly." All gradations are lost and the concept of age becomes an artificial product of the way in which the real ages are collapsed into the categories. Obviously, there is not much to recommend purposive loss of information in this manner. Fortunately, some scholars understand the problem and are making strides in resolving some of the operationalization concerns. As a good example, recent work in gender roles promises to move the treatment of "sex" beyond its usual nominal, and dichotomous, categorization (see for instance, Lorber, 1996), but there is little which suggests a similar understanding of race or age.

Disinterest

The problem of poor conceptualization is supported by a seemingly general disinterest in the adequacy of our measurements. Blalock (1982:8), for instance, has noted that sociology and political science have failed to pay attention to conceptualization and measurement to the same degree that economics and psychology have. He attributes this to an inability to experiment with social structures, the complexity of the subject matter, a lack of resources, and the problems associated with indirect measurement. Whatever the reasons, criminologists have rarely made attempts to establish the reliability and validity of their concepts (Huizinga and Elliott [1987] are a notable exception to this statement). On the other hand, our research designs inevitably include a commentary on their external validity (we may not know *what* we are generalizing, but whatever it is, it is indeed representative). It may be that a by-product of the sociological desire to discuss *rates* of phenomena is that external validity issues will always take precedence over internal ones.

Difficulty of Measurement

A final rationale used to perpetuate current conceptions of race, gender, and age is that these basic sociological concepts are difficult to measure. Under this approach a close, but simple, approximation is preferable to the (assumed) elaborate methodology needed to measure a complex concept. If that approximation can also serve to measure other concepts, then so much the better. While I have no objection to this position as a first-stage form of measurement, one has to ask when the time will come to drop the use of proxies and attempt more difficult, but more rewarding, measurement schemes.

The chief problem here is that a simple approximation cannot be used to examine the nuances of relationships. Interpretation of complex effects is impossible as is the examination of relationships with other concepts in a theoretical network. When an approximation represents several concepts, problems of interaction among the associated concepts are also masked and cannot be investigated. Other problems are multiplied as well.

Difficulty in measuring concepts should not serve as a barrier when those concepts are basic to a discipline's subject matter. At the least, criminologists (or sociologists) should develop independent measures of the various dimensions approximated by race and gender and include them in our research designs. Even if we cannot locate the majority of them, it should not be too difficult to incorporate a few of these basic dimensions. Other, equally difficult, concepts have been elaborated by other disciplines, with various dimensions separated and measurement scales created. Only in this fashion can estimations be made of the effect of various social statuses and roles on criminality.

THE LINK BETWEEN CONCEPTS, MEASUREMENT AND THEORY

While this may oversimplify, the current overemphasis on quantitative empiricism is even dangerous for measurement. The problem has to do with the way in which we develop knowledge. Theorizing and theory construction are supposed to be based on existing empirical evidence. Yet, how do we achieve empirical evidence? The obvious answer is that evidence is derived from measurement. Now for the second question: How do we measure? The answer to that question is by developing measuring instruments. Those instruments are limited by our ability to measure—our techniques and skills—not the images we can imagine. Measurement, then, is technique based rather than creative. If so, empirical knowledge is limited by technique as well and a tautology arises. Empirical theories contain what we already know and merely attempt to achieve new ways to reconstruct the relationships. *There is no room left for creativity and imagination.* Under such perspectives our major theoretical task becomes that of finding new ways to measure existing ideas.

Concepts and Measurement

The notion of empirical measurement is also important for reasons of superficiality. Any concept is more complex than its measurement. Indeed, a concept is nothing more than an abstract representation of some piece of reality (or imagined reality). Any variable, on the other hand, is a singular, measurable piece of that abstraction. It takes several variables to capture even the most simplistic concept, yet none of those variables, in and of themselves, truly represent the concept. Thus, even a simplistic concept can be misrepresented in its whole.

To illustrate this point, let us first use an example that is noncontroversial and noncriminological: a ball that is completely uniform in all respects. Its surface is equally smooth in all places, its diameter never changes, and its composition is the same throughout. If the ball is conceived as a concept, then the task is to measure the concept in such a way that we find the essence of the ball. Now imagine a needle as the measuring instrument. We can take the needle and stick it into any part of the ball and where it sticks we may take that area of the ball as representative of the entire ball. We shall even make the needle a reliable instrument by devising a mechanical holder for the needle that does not deviate as it is moved toward the ball. Now we stick the needle into the ball and conclude from that specific evidence what the ball is like. Indeed, because of its uniformity, any area of the ball would be the same; thus, all evidence and all conclusions would be the same. Yet how do we know the shape of the object?

Now we introduce some degree of complexity. Imagine a baseball. It is composed of a core around which string is wound and then a rawhide cover is stitched on. We now jab the needle into the ball, hitting the stitching. Thus, with no more measurements we conclude the ball is a stitch of thread. But you may protest that one measurement surely doesn't suffice, and you would be correct: science repeats its measurements. Using the same "instrument," we stick the ball again, and again we hit the thread. Why is this so? It is because the instrument is a reliable one—always hitting the ball at the same place and from the same angle. This particular problem will exist until the measuring instrument is changed—and then researchers will fight among themselves about which instrument is better and what the ball is composed of.

Returning to the criminological realm, a similar concept might be a "broken home." Assuming that broken homes are related to juvenile delinquency, one might be interested in operationalizing the concept. The first task is to stick the needle into the concept, that is, to create a measuring instrument. Unfortunately, there are probably no uniform concepts in the social world, thus complexity is a given. *Where* we stick the needle (measuring instrument) becomes critical to the representation of broken homes. In the previous analogy, one might end up measuring the seams rather than the dominant part of the concept. Thus, we quibble and argue about whether broken homes constitute a "single-family home," one in which a "father" is absent, or one in which the parents are somehow separated but not through death. Yet none of these measures may actually represent the dominant part of the concept of a broken home. If an intact home has a problem parent (assume for instance an alcoholic parent), a "non-broken" home may actually be a worse environment for a juvenile. It is possible that the quality of parenting (or whatever constitutes the *essence*) of a broken home is actually *enhanced* by the departure of a parent. Therefore, several questions need to be asked about the concept, and at least one needs to be answered: Is a "broken home" another way of saying that the home "environment" is inadequate? In short, is one concept merely a subconcept of another? If so, what and how should we measure?

Variables and Theory

While operationalization is an important issue for measurement of concepts, the relative simplicity of the examples above obscures a potentially larger problem: the *dimension* of examination. This is as crucial, if not more so, than the measuring instrument used. Dimension of examination has to do with the direction from which measurement is undertaken. If one persists in understanding broken homes as merely the absence of a parent, the concept is measured unidimensionally, that is, in one dimension only. Because most concepts are complex, it stands to reason that a measurement scheme will tend toward unidimensionality. In that event researchers may persist in potentially erroneous measurement (even with great reliability) that either wrongly supports the concept or discourages other research. Clearly, from this viewpoint, it is better to triangulate measurements of a concept (i.e., create multiple and different measurements). Moreover, it is also advantageous to bring multiple methodologies to bear on a concept (e.g., supplement survey research with observational design and experiment). It is a fact that stronger confidence can be placed in results when multiple dimensions of measurement are used by a researcher.

It is important to understand that empirical evidence can be tantamount to a variable purporting to represent a concept when that is never actually the case. As long as the same measurement is made with the same instrument and from the same dimension, the "evidence" will appear strong, yet it will be misleading. This is a crucial point because we do not use variables in theory—we use *concepts*.[9] And those concepts are tied to the reality we see about us. Thus, any theory derived entirely from evidence may never come close to representing reality. And, at the same time, such a theory may be empirically supported and replicable. The task is to make sure that reality is of primary concern. Here, then, lies the real danger of conducting analyses that use secondary data as proxy measures of theoretical concepts.

CONCLUSIONS

We need better measurement tempered with an understanding of the world around us—not mere technological expertise. We need to undertake a serious examination of all of our concepts but particularly our basic ones: crime, criminals, and our critical explanatory variables. That has been sorely lacking.

In a nutshell, I am claiming that a conceptual stagnation is inherent within the commonly accepted criminological definition of crime and the modes of measurement commonly used for critical variables. This circumstance obviates a real examination of criminal behavior, fosters a myopic view of crime, and creates a politically based discipline. We must begin to expand both our reason and our discipline. Doing this requires that criminologists turn their attention to forms of social harm (i.e., that which is not legally "crime") while remaining sensitive to the conditions that engender legality. In short, we must be able to explain harmful *behavior*, whether or not it falls within the legal rubric of crime.

I have also attempted to point out the fallacy of oversimplifying measurement of our concepts. I do not deny that the three variables discussed here are highly correlated with crime; in fact, these variables were chosen for that very reason. Nonetheless, to assume that the simplified variables are *actual* causal agents is entirely another matter. Such a fiction is at best misleading and at worst keeps criminologists from a true, accurate, understanding of their subject matter.

There are also implications for theory here. Criminologists have been searching for causal agents among the various structures and institutions of society, while at the same time introducing gender, race, and age as control variables in our research on those theories. If, in fact, these variables serve as approximations of various social roles and statuses, social structure becomes a redundant explanation. By separating the various concepts as has been suggested here, interrelations may become apparent and current theoretical models might be respecified. These comments may also help to explain why some of our theories seem to represent intuitive reality and yet find little empirical support.

Finally, I am also attempting to encourage a movement toward complexity in our conceptualizing. A failure to consider concepts or the use of simpler surrogate variables because of assumed difficulty in measurement is no longer appropriate. Recent understandings of causality, especially those which are probabilistic in nature, point to greater complexity in causal explanation. Criminology (and the social sciences in general) cannot afford to continue to embrace simplicity at the cost of losing the essence of what is being measured.

NOTES

1. Portions of this chapter were originally written with the assistance of Marilyn McShane and presented in a paper at the 1994 meetings of the Pacific Sociological Association.

2. I realize that crime is technically a legal category of behavior, defined by the criminal statutes of a political body. For some criminologists (social reaction theorists, anarchists, radicals), this has been exactly the point of contention. My concern is that legal "crime" is relative and, thus, constrains the

nature of the primary criminological dependent variable with different political visions in time and space.

3. The issue may be even larger. Jeff Walker argues forcibly that there is no measurement theory in criminology.

4. Recently, some funding has been available to "crime theory." In comparison to the money being spent on the system, however, it remains negligible.

5. There is, of course, an entire branch of "non-mainstream" criminology characterized by various terminologies ("critical," "radical," "left realist," "postmodern," and "constitutive") that has championed various approaches to nonlegal definitions of crime.

6. Thus it is not biological sex itself that becomes important, but the culturally ascribed and imputed roles associated with sex or, put more succinctly, the "gender" of the person.

7. This is the point of departure for better measurement of race (and age, gender, and social class). The concept of race should first be broken down into its various cultural imputations and then those should be operationalized as variables measuring concrete characteristics. While the ideas above may prove useful, I leave this task of developing these measures to social scientists more familiar with the topic.

8. This quest to reduce explanation to a few important variables also raises a question about the quest itself. Because we refer to correlations as "explaining" variance, it is likely the case that explanation has sometimes become nothing more than significant correlations. Thus, statistical explanation has become intermingled with substance explanation. A second problem is that parsimony fuels the emphasis on linear models. There are nonlinear analytical tools available that are capable of dealing with complexity. Many of these have been recently developed as a product of chaos-theory-based interest in modeling highly complex systems.

9. This very fact may help to explain why theories are difficult to test. The theorist is not normally concerned with variables. In order to translate a theory for empirical testing, the richness of the theory must be abandoned for objective simplicity. Because of this, there is some question as to whether any but the most simplistic theory is *capable* of being adequately represented by variables.

REFERENCES

Ball, Richard A., and G. David Curry (1995). The logic of definition in criminology: Purposes and methods for defining "gangs." *Criminology* 33: 225–245.

Barak, Greg (1995). *Integrating Criminologies*. Boston, MA: Allyn and Bacon.

Becker, Howard S. (1963). *Outsiders: Studies in the Sociology of Deviance*. New York, NY: Free Press.

Blalock, Hubert (1982). *Measurement and Conceptualization in the Social Sciences*. Beverly Hills, Sage.

Gottfredson, Michael, and Travis Hirschi (1990). *A General Theory of Crime*. Palo Alto, CA: Stanford University Press.

Hughes, Everett C. (1945). Dilemmas and contradictions of status. *American Journal of Sociology* 50: 353–359.

Huizinga, David and Delbert S. Elliott (1987). Juvenile offenders: Prevalence, offender incidence, and arrest rates by race. *Crime and Delinquency* 33: 206–223.

Lorber, Judith (1996). Beyond the binaries: Depolarizing the categories of sex, sexuality, and gender. *Sociological Inquiry* 66: 143–159.

Lynd, Robert S. and Helen M. (1937). *Middletown in Transition: A Study in Cultural Conflicts*. New York, NY: Harcourt, Brace.

Sampson, Robert J., and John H. Laub (1993). *Crime in the Making: Pathways and Turning Points through Life*. Cambridge, MA: Harvard University Press.

Schwendinger, Herman and Julia (1970). Defenders of order or guardians of human rights? *Issues in Criminology* 7: 72-81.

Selltiz, Claire, Lawrence S. Wrightsman, and Stuart W. Cook (1976). *Research Methods in Social Relations*, 3rd ed. New York, NY: Holt, Rinehart and Winston.

Simpson, Sally (1991). Caste, class, and violent crime: Explaining differences in female offending. *Criminology* 29: 115–36.

Smart, Carol (1995). *Law, Crime and Sexuality: Essays in Feminism*. London: Sage.

Stevens, S.S. (1946). On the theory of scales of measurement. *Science* 103(2684): 677–680.

Sutherland, Edwin H. (1945). Is white-collar crime "crime?" *American Sociological Review* 10: 132–139.

Tappan, Paul W. (1947). Who is the criminal? *American Sociological Review* 12: 96–102.

Wilkins, Leslie T. (1968). Offense patterns. *International Encyclopedia of the Social Sciences* 3:476–483

Wilson, James Q. (1982). *Thinking about Crime*, 2nd ed. New York, NY: Basic Books.

Wilson, James Q., and Richard J. Herrnstein (1985). *Crime and Human Nature: The Definitive Study of the Causes of Crime.* New York, NY: Simon and Schuster.

CHAPTER FIVE

The Search for Reality

INTRODUCTION

I have long had the nagging feeling that most criminological theories lack a real feel for the human condition and for the complexity of life. Our theories variously paint a picture of criminals who had too many bad friends, or who were under too much pressure to succeed, or who were not given the proper values as a child. While we can all nod our heads sagely and say "those indeed are the critical variables of criminality," most of us do not really believe that. Humans are too complex to be affected so simply, and *not one of the theorists and researchers would attribute his or her own behavior to something so simple.* Where is a picture of the excitement, the pump of adrenaline, the breathlessness, we know from our own small transgressions? Existing theory is dangerously *sterile*; life is not.

CRIMINOLOGISTS AS "TREETOP FLIERS"

I believe theory is sterile because, by and large, criminologists have moved to a comfortable level of abstraction that allows them to see crime and criminals as part of the social structure, or part of social classes, or, failing that, as part of social groups. How else do we explain a discipline primarily studying its subjects through data collected by and for governmental agencies? Based on years of discussions with my colleagues, it seems to be sadly true that many of them have rarely seen and talked with a real criminal, much less actually studied such a person. But, the argument goes, sociologically based criminology is properly doing what it is supposed to: study aggregates in society.

If criminology is to be merely sociological, then we have a problem because no one is studying the real people. In a wonderful turn of phrase, Mark Hamm (1996:525) has called such researchers and theorists "treetop fliers," people who skim over the top of the subject as if they were in a helicopter, never landing to see what is down below and thereby getting their shoes dirty. There are, of course, some people in the trenches, so to speak — but the level of abstraction in the dominant approach tends to keep us from seeing a reality other than the one constructed by our social data. Having discussed conceptualization, I will now probe the problems of current, positivistically oriented, quantitative methodology.

THE META-PARADIGM OF QUANTITATIVE METHODOLOGY

If one cannot find paradigms in theoretical development, surely one may find them in methodology. Indeed, one may argue even more forcefully for the existence of evidence-gathering paradigms. Different areas of inquiry clearly emphasize certain methodologies. For example, those studying the drug-crime relationship primarily engage in surveys that ask drug users about their habits;[1] victimologists survey victims (the National Crime Panel) about their experiences, and questions about crime are frequently answered with official data (the UCR). Rarely do the drugs and crime researchers use data such as emergency room records or insurance records, and victimologists do not ask criminals about their victims. I am not arguing here that *no* researcher steps outside of the paradigm, just that most of the information comes from a single methodology. Any overemphasis of a single approach is dangerous for knowledge. Just as it serves well to triangulate measurements when attempting to capture a phenomenon, so does triangulation of methods serve us. If one finds the same thing in both quantitative and qualitative examinations, the evidence for the existence of that thing would be even more compelling.

Lack of Substance

It would seem to be a truism that our methods of determining the existence of things are questionable. That this is so, in any time and in any place, is rather easy to demonstrate. Imagine what today's researchers would say about knowledge-gaining approaches of 500 years ago, or even a century ago. The people of that age believed just as we do today that they were discovering eternal truths. Yet those truths, yesterday's and today's, are not the same. *Our* truths are real, yesterday's were not. The fact is that today's "truth" is no different from yesteryear's in one crucial respect—it is a product of existing methodology and perspective. Thus, tomorrow's knowledge-producers will laugh at today's pronouncements of reality.

Reality and Perception

There is another important facet in this time-sensitive example. Truth is a product of existing techniques of evidence production. One does not "know" reality beyond one's ability to test that reality. How, for instance, would Newton have been able to convince people of his theory of gravity prior to evidence techniques of experimentation and advanced mathematics? How would Einstein's theory of relativity have fared even in Newton's day? In short, *accepted* reality and truth is time-specific, not eternal. Humans probably will never know truth and reality, primarily because we must first *perceive* it, and that brings into play all our biases and methodologies. Rather than directly seeking truth, perhaps a better approach is to ask what we would be happy with, what would be useful to us?

A Statistical Reality

What, then, is the substance of criminological reality? I believe it is primarily a mathematical, statistical substance that owes its origins to the collection of social statistics begun in the 1930s in the U.S. We do not actually deal with criminals themselves, instead we count them and classify their acts. This reality is a mathematical one because it is based on rates of behaviors, indices of social variables, and averages. These have little substance beyond the numbers that produce them. But, a counter-argument would point out, these are all based on *real* individual behaviors and characteristics and numbers of items; and that I do not deny. Nonetheless, once each of these is enumerated and aggregated, the individual is lost and the substance of the new reality is an aggregate construct.

Statistical analysis requires the use of numbers to represent concepts. This representation is based on a logic system—mathematics—invented by humans in order to better understand the world. Once we change reality into numbers and process those numbers with mathematical statements, we "understand" reality better. But exactly *what* reality do we understand better? The process requires that we first conceptualize reality. This is not a unique problem for statistical analysis, indeed conceptualization is the one ubiquitous problem and the basic source of error. It is the attempt to further represent reality by operationalizing the original concepts that introduces a second-order problem. Thus by attempting to find a way to concretely express what we think we see, a secondary representation of reality takes place and a second form of error is introduced. But statistical analysis does not stop here—a third form of representation and potential error is established. That is when a measuring instrument is created so that numbers may be produced or when a "variable" is measured. The way we measure becomes critical. If any part of the variable is improperly measured, error (separation from reality) creeps in. Actually, the mere translation *into* numbers yields one more schism between reality and interpretation. A fourth source of error is derived from violations of the assumptions of statistical techniques and misunderstandings about the shape of the data. Each statistic was based on certain assumptions when it was created. In many cases the assumptions were not discussed, they existed because the statistic was created to work with a certain analytical problem. Unfortunately, the more sophisticated statistics require a greater number of assumptions about the data. Because virtually no set of data exactly matches an assumed distribution, it is a safe statement that nearly all statistical analyses have assumption violations and, therefore, some degree of unknown error. And a fifth order of error comes into play when one attempts to interpret the results of the analysis. Two of these orders of error are unavoidable in any case: we must conceptualize and interpret regardless of method. What should be clear, however, is that interpreted statistical reality is five orders removed from the original phenomenon. It is foolhardy to claim that statistically related techniques provide a better grasp of reality—they simply provide *another* view of reality.

Analytical techniques fail when they oversimplify the world, just as theories do. Deciding what research method and analytical tool we will use is merely another way of asking "How will we view reality?" The assumption of our present random-distribution-based (stochastic) statistics is that if certain forms of systematic observations are not present in data, then the results are random and nothing is happening. This I shall discuss in detail as the core of Chapters six and seven. Similarly, we prefer orderly, systematic causes that are as close in time to the presumed effect as possible. This shows a preference for a nice, neat universe that flows along human logic patterns. While this form of logic obviously served humans (and other organisms) well in our biological past by keeping us from eating poison berries and foods, it is certainly not the logic of a complex universe. Other than the fact that it is evolutionarily ingrained, why should we continue to use such logic as a primary way of knowing the world about us?

Aggregate Realities

We have made another critical decision about viewing reality. Information is routinely collected by aggregate methods. Even when we collect information from individuals, it is combined and aggregated. In short, individuals are not to be trusted—but aggregate information from individuals somehow becomes truth. Yet is it those individuals who *live* in a rich, complex reality. Aggregated reality is a *constructed*, abstract and simpler reality. It is methodology that contributes to this state of affairs, and there are two ways in which that happens.

The favored method of the social sciences in general and criminology in particular is the survey, whether in interview or questionnaire format.[2] This technique is expressly designed for the analysis of information about groups and probably became popular during the 1930s as a result of criminology (as part of sociology) moving away from individual modes of analysis and toward the analysis of classes and groups.

Statistical analysis also contributes to the aggregated-methodology hegemony. An individual is simply not a "statistical entity." Because most of our analytical techniques are based on stochastic methods, large samples are normally required to distinguish real effects from random error. Thus, not only is the individual ignored but so, too, are small groups. As a result most of our discoveries and solutions pertain to an abstract reality. In short, our evidence sheds little light on what individuals do and why they do it, but we know quite a bit about artificial groups.

This problem even extends beyond the nature of groups. National data have been used to reconstitute cities, areas, and neighborhoods. The concept of neighborhoods yields an excellent example. Theoretical constructions of neighborhood have focused on social and environmental factors within a particular geographic boundary. More to the point, theorists discuss the places where groups of people live and the way in which they relate to each other. The sampling technique employed in national samples does not allow for the interviewing of a neighborhood area, nor does it enable the reconstruction of the neighborhood concept. Constructing and characterizing neighborhoods through the use of variables in those samples cannot possibly result in a *real* neighborhood, instead the technique creates an artificial neighborhood. That is, the "neighborhood" will be comprised of interviewees from similar environments across the nation *but not the same neighborhood.* Depending on the techniques with which this hypothetical neighborhood is built, the "neighbors" will either share single variables, which may be independent of each other, or constellations of variables which produce clusters of similar "neighbors." Even in the later case, however, there is no reason to believe that those sharing a cluster also share the values and social environment that constitute the essence of a sociological neighborhood. In short, national probability samples do not, and cannot, create real neighborhoods but they do create an abstract, statistical neighborhood.

The Requirement of A Priori Evidence

The position that theory needs to be based on evidence and then subsequently supported by evidence is commonplace. An examination of the theory-evidence relationship, however, suggests that it is more complex than it seems and, at least in part, based on ideological assumptions. First, if we must have evidence of something in order to theorize about it, then we will never be capable of thinking of more than our evidence-gathering methodologies allow. Independent thought, intuitive reasoning, and imagination will never be allowed to suggest *what might be.* In order to have theoretical concepts, a measuring instrument must be available and have produced information. Thus, we must have thought of a need and thereby invented the measuring instrument. But, if evidence cannot come before the measuring instrument, how did we know we needed to create it? A tautology begins to emerge in the rationale.

Such positions also ignore the history of science. They assume that evidence always provides information for advances in thought, otherwise referred to as the "building block" theory of science. Kuhn (1970) and Lakatos (1970), among others, have shown this view to be generally false. Indeed, it appears that leaps of intuition and ignorance of standing positions have been more likely to produce breakthroughs. These are *not* necessarily evidence-derived solutions to problems. Thus, it would be a grave mistake to limit ourselves to evidence-derived thought and theories. However, it *would* be comfortable for those invested in the status quo.

A second part of the evidence-theory relationship concerns the use of databases to create theory, otherwise known as "grounded" theory or "empirical" theory. Theories are composed of two pieces: the nomological network of concepts that constitute the theoretical relationships and the specifics derived from the network (the empirical statements). It should be kept in mind that the latter are predicated on the former, but not vice versa. That is, empirical statements serve as a single way to represent only one of the network of theoretical relationships—it is not possible to reconstruct a body from one of its atoms. Moreover, the empirical statement is only one way of interpreting the network. When a database is plumbed for empirical relationships (the method of constructing grounded theories), one is essentially taking that single interpretation (or perhaps several of the single interpretations) and attempting to "explain" it. This is done through constructing a "theory" that contains the relationship or, in short, inferring the nomological network. This is simply not possible. Indeed, it is an attempt to substitute explanation for understanding. Moreover, it is replete with ideological contamination. For example, previous examinations of the characteristics of prisoners have led to explanations of criminality (see the works of Lombroso, Goddard, Goring, and Hooton for excellent examples). There is simply no way in which to interpret these observed relationships except in a pre-existing belief system.

All of this, of course, assumes that the "relationships" were not a product of measurement error. Independently, even if the relationships are true, how are they to be falsified? Only a theory which rises above *a priori* empirical evidence can be falsified by empirical evidence. As a final issue for grounded theory, they lack power and utility because anomalies easily destroy them. Evidence that is contrary to the database-specific evidence which served to establish the theory is generally not explainable. When evidence anomalies cannot be explained and incorporated, theories do not survive long.

Understanding Error

For those who would maintain the dominance of quantitative methodology, there is one remaining issue to cover. Even though the essence of research and analysis is estimating error, an examination of published materials indicates that we have little appreciation of that fact. By this I mean that both methodology and statistics are devoted to identifying variance, partitioning that variance, and eliminating (or controlling) error variance. Indeed, there is little else that statistics, particularly stochastically-based statistics, do. Yet it is clear from a perusal of the journal literature that not only is error rarely discussed, but even when mentioned, it is given short shrift with comments such as, "It is evident that, whatever error exists in our analyses, the thrust of the data are clearly more important in scope." Frankly, it is not "evident" in most cases because neither the researcher not the reader has enough information to assess the amount and effect of error. This is particularly so in the common case of probability statistics used without benefit of random samples. It needs to be understood that estimates of error are important; without them we have little evidence to presume that our data inferences are reasonable.

PERSPECTIVES AND VALUES:
THE SUBJECTIVITY/OBJECTIVITY CONUNDRUM

Subjectivity is not necessarily the antithesis of objectivity, at least as we practice it in the social sciences (see Groves and Lynch [1990] for an excellent discussion of this point). Objectivity requires that we do not interject our *own* biases into the interpretation of phenomena. It does *not* require that we ignore the subjective interpretations of others. Indeed, the subjective views of others make up the subject matter of the social and behavioral sciences. This section deals with the ways in which an appreciation of subjectivity has been subverted or devalued.

Devaluing the Perspective of the Actor

One form of subjectivity places value on the perspective of the actor, what the actor sees and believes about his or her social and natural reality. The old Chicago School understood this subjectivity and its importance in understanding people, tempering both method and theory with descriptions of actors' lives in their own words (c.f., the life histories and ecological studies written by Anderson [1923], Shaw [1930], Sutherland [1937], and Zorbaugh [1929]). Matza (1969) even argued that the very essence of the Chicago School was this understanding and appreciation of subjectivity in the deviants they studied.

W. I. Thomas's famous dictum that one acts on the basis of what one *believes* to be true reflects the general position of early criminology. Somewhere along the line, criminologists seem to have filed this as an interesting observation and decided to ignore its implications. Yet it is a powerful influence in human life. For instance, even though there is no objective, rational reason, many individuals are scared of the dark—and act accordingly. Without knowing of such a belief, a researcher would be hard pressed to locate the motivation for such behavior in the objective environment. Indeed, because people act according to what they *think* is true, objective reality may be immaterial. Thus, there are at least two realities for any actor, the subjective and the objective. Because the objective reality first must be perceived in order to come into play, the subjective reality may be of greater value for predicting behavior.

Devaluing Experience

A second problem created by social science objectivity is that experience is devalued. The actor is given credit only for personalized experiences, which lack systematic and rigorous observations, a necessity in the empirical world of science. This is an intriguing phenomenon, for social scientists do not deny their own experiences. It is not uncommon to hear criminologists talk proudly of their experiences in the field and in the research process (and other personal experiences, as well). Indeed, they not only admit the use of those experiences, but value them. Such experiences help the criminologist correctly perceive important factors and properly interpret data. Researchers learn their trade in part through education and in part through the trial and error of experience. The latter is particularly important in learning how to adjust the idealized research designs of the classroom to the reality of the field. Criminal justice scholars have taken the position that field experience is so important that one cannot relate to the subject matter without it, and certainly one cannot teach well without it. All this is well and good, but where is the objective evidence that the information gained from such experience is gathered in a systematic and rigorous fashion and therefore "better" than the experience of subjects? It simply does not exist. To validate one is to validate the other; to negate one is to negate the other.

The Perspective of the Researcher

It seems that social scientists have devalued the actor's subjectivity in a chase for scientific objectivity. In truth, by devaluing the perspective of the actor, social science has actually introduced bias into observations. Indeed, the rejection of the actor's perspective has been justified chiefly by a belief that the actor does not know what his or her motivations actually are, that any explanations given for behavior are actually rationalizations. Where behavior is concerned, the social scientist knows best. The one person without bias, with no danger of falling into subjectivity, and coldly analytical is the researcher. This hubris may well be the most dangerous error that a researcher can make.

Finally, where is the evidence that social scientists actually know what their subjects (criminals, victims, and criminal justice workers) are actually thinking and doing? How they actually live? In truth, it is more likely that criminologists are well experienced with large datasets on these subjects, that they know what the computers are doing, and that they know the reality of statistics. But do these things actually constitute the subjects? Certainly not. As a result, the experiences of a good number of criminologists assist in interpretation of their subject matter (the data) but not their subjects.

Language and Constructed Reality

A final subjectivity concern is expressed by language. Postmodern scholars have referred to this as a form of "privileging discourse" (see Arrigo [1996]; Milovanovic [1993, 1994]). Researchers' use of terms such as "subjects" serve to detach actors from their social reality and demean their subjective interpretations. By constructing research terms in an atmosphere that values objectivity, the subtle implications of using those terms validates the very valuing. I suspect the use of numbers itself is a very powerful piece of this overall conundrum. *Nothing* is more devoid of feeling and subjectivity than representing thoughts, feelings, actions, and actors as numbers. Thus, a new reality is constructed by the use of abstract concepts and measurements designed around the idea of objectivity. The problem right now is that quantitative methodology represents the master signifier in social science and thereby delegitimizes all qualitative discourse.

CONCLUSION

Because I cannot see truth any better than the next person, I have no final answers to the problems discussed in this and previous chapters. Being concerned with methodological and analytical paradigms in criminology and criminal justice and increasing attention to measurement does not represent a panacea for the problems. Indeed, too much attention runs the risk of overemphasizing technique at the expense of conceptualization. I certainly do not want to see the field rush into a position that the essence of a phenomenon is that which is measured. Indeed, I have argued that measurement, no matter how well done, is still an approximation of a phenomenon, not the phenomenon itself. I believe that existing mainstream approaches are virtually bankrupt in their ability to tell us much about crime and criminality. We desperately need a new paradigm or new perspectives by which to view our subject.

So what can we do? In the main, I propose that we facilitate "criminology of the edge"—a criminology that appreciates the complexity of life, the seeming chaos of rational and irrational action, and couched within a subjective understanding. This does not mean that we must cast off all that we now do. There is value in carefully and systematically analyzing data. We will, however, have to appreciate the value of relativism in order to understand motivation from the point of view of individual actors (not from the point of view of researchers, as we do now). And, most of all, we need to think more about the *feel* of life: the pleasure of action and the excitement of the edge. Thus, researchers need to devote more time to being in the field, directly observing subjects, talking with subjects and, most of all, *understanding* subjects. If we take this perspective and value such versions of knowledge, it just may be that we come to know more—surely we will know *differently* (see two recent articles by John Braithwaite [1993, 1996]). If we fail to do something different than we are doing today, I believe many of us will be reminded of the existential and poignant line from a Peggy Lee song of the 1960s: "Is this all there is?"

Instead of a new *theory*, I believe what we really need is a new *metatheory*, a more instructive way of perceiving and examining reality. Certainly, that is one of the major messages of postmodernists. There are alternative forms of knowing and creating evidence. We usually see two alternatives: "objective" and quantitative evidence, or "subjective" and qualitative evidence. These two need to be used in complementary rather than exclusive fashion. Yet, the quantitative age may have reached its culmination. The question of *what* to study and *how* to perceive it may now lie mostly within the domain of the qualitative. In short, quantitative methodology *needs* the assistance of qualitative methodology.

NOTES

1. Actually, there is an entire data collection effort known as the Drug Use Forecasting system (DUF). Data are collected in 23 cities by interviewing arrestees and detainees and by gathering urine samples. Strangely, this effort seems to have spawned entirely new criteria for surveys, including voluntary participation, letting the interviewers determine who they want to interview, and representing quarterly arrests by a quota of 225 interviews done at one time. While this survey approach is the embodiment of poor methodology, the worst aspect is that data are not collected to test any hypotheses nor may they be used to support any theory. Indeed, DUF is an excellent example of data for data's sake.

2. This expressly ignores the analysis of secondary data, which is probably the most frequently used methodological approach. Virtually all of the data used in this method are aggregated.

REFERENCES

Anderson, Nels (1923). *The Hobo*. Chicago, IL: University of Chicago Press.

Arrigo, Bruce (1996). *The Contours of Psychiatric Justice: A Postmodern Critique of Mental Illness, Criminal Insanity, and the Law*. New York, NY: Garland.

Braithwaite, John (1993). Beyond positivism: Learning from contextual integrated strategies. *Journal of Research in Crime and Delinquency* 30: 383–399.

Braithwaite, John (1996). Searching for epistemologically plural criminology (and finding some). *Australian and New Zealand Journal of Criminology* 29: 142–146.

Groves, W. Byron, and Michael J. Lynch (1990). Reconciling structural and subjective approaches to the study of crime. *Journal of Research in Crime and Delinquency* 27: 348–375.

Hamm, Mark (1996). Book review of Zimring and Hawkins' *Incapacitation: Penal Confinement and the Restraint of Crime. Justice Quarterly* 13(3): 525–530.

Kuhn, Thomas (1970). *The Structure of Scientific Revolutions*, 2nd ed., enlarged. Chicago, IL: University of Chicago Press.

Lakatos, Imre (1970). Falsification and the methodology of scientific research programmes. In I. Lakatos and A. Musgrave (eds.) *Criticism and the Growth of Knowledge*. Cambridge, UK: Cambridge University Press.

Matza, David (1969). *Becoming Deviant*. Englewood Cliffs, NJ: Prentice Hall.

Milovanovic, Dragan (1993). Borromean knots and the constitution of sense in juridico-discursive production. *Legal Studies Forum* 17: 171–192.

Milovanovic, Dragan (1994). The decentered subject in law: Contributions of topology, psychoanalytic semiotics and chaos theory. *Studies in Psychoanalytic Theory* 3: 93–127.

Shaw, Clifford R. (1930). *The Jackroller*. Chicago, IL: University of Chicago Press.

Stevens, S.S. (1946). On scales of measurement. *Science* 103(2684): 677–680.

Sutherland, Edwin H. (1937). *The Professional Thief*. Chicago, IL: University of Chicago Press.

Zorbaugh, Harvey W. (1929). *The Gold Coast and the Slum*. Chicago, IL: University of Chicago Press.

CHAPTER SIX

Chaos, Complex Systems, and Self-Organized Criticality[1]

THE NEED FOR A NEW METATHEORY

The critical need for criminology, and social science in general, is to achieve a better understanding of the complexity of reality. As the previous arguments have shown, the dominant perspectives of the past three decades have produced a rather simplified and primarily sociological version of reality. I have also argued that one of the major reasons for this state of affairs is the mode of evidence production. Clearly, a new paradigm of evidence production is necessary as is a new metatheory that incorporates a complex reality.

What ingredients should this new metatheory have? As Chapter two demonstrated, recent research and theorizing has located a few new concepts that, taken together, promise a new slant on criminological reality. First, we now have evidence that *change* is important to behavioral events and criminological variables (Sampson and Laub, 1993). Second, we have acknowledged that crime is merely one of an *analogous* set of behaviors (Gottfredson and Hirschi, 1990). Third, there is now sufficient evidence that crime and associated phenomena often behave in a *nonlinear* fashion. Finally, physicists, mathematicians and others have developed sufficient evidence that many phenomena behave *chaotically*.[2] Taken together, these four pieces of a "new" criminological reality are revolutionary; they suggest a dynamic, complex, multidimensional, and even subjective social reality. Such a reality is not really surprising, indeed, it smacks of the observations made by recent qualitative criminologists (Katz, 1988; Ferrell, 1993) and can even be seen in the work of the old Chicago School (Shaw, 1930; Anderson, 1923).

THEORETICAL MODELS CAPABLE OF COMPLEXITY

How do we get to such a theoretical reality? The problems discussed in previous chapters are critical to the type and form of theory construction in criminology. In the face of an assumption that the social world is complex and subjective, the underlying metatheoretical assumptions of existing theories lend themselves to the construction of simplistic systems. Granted, it is easier to interpret parsimonious relationships than complex ones, but ease of interpretation does not constitute ease of understanding. Complex systems demand theoretical systems capable of explaining that complexity.

Recent developments in theoretical physics, particularly chaos theory with its work on highly complex problems, promise some insight into methods of constructing more capable criminological theories. The concepts of chaos theory suggest that understanding of ultra-complex systems may be reduced by (a) dimension of examination and (b) evidence-producing tools. By dimension of examination, I mean that an apparent randomly-ordered system may yield patterns only under certain levels of examination or under certain modes of observing the phenomena. In a simplistic example, a two-dimensional plot of data may be viewed as fully random until depth is added and the plot rotated. At that point, and from that dimension of examination, fully systematic relationships may be located.

Evidence-producing tools imply similar problems. All evidence is produced by some particular form of observation. A critical point about observation is that when something is observed, assumptions about its nature are made. Observations cannot, by themselves, yield the totality of any phenomenon; therefore, the form of observation carries with it differential views of reality. Thus, evidence-producing tools rely on implicit assumptions about what will be considered evidence and about what will *not* be. As an example, ordinary statistical tools based on stochastic[3] probability distributions require that variables be systematically present, and systematically correlated, or else they are assumed to be random and non-causal. In the example of the two-dimensional plot above, a bivariate statistical tool will find no correlation; on the other hand, a multivariate stochastic tool might. If the plot is expanded to a dynamic series over time, where an event occurs systematically, but under multi-specified infrequent conditions, even a multivariate stochastic tool will identify the result as random. As a result, stochastic statistics will be ill suited for locating non-proximate patterns among such variables and data and will therefore, at best, find only low correlations.

How, then, do we incorporate multiple dimensions and high degrees of complexity into criminological theory? Some criminologists (Milovanovic [1994, 1996, 1997a, 1997b]; Pepinsky [1991]; Vila [1994]; Walker [1996]; Young [1991, 1997]) have already used chaos theory as a method of producing insights into crime and criminal behavior. All of these writers have seen the general chaos perspective as a way to locate new patterns in existing realities. Before moving to a simplified history and explanation of chaos theory, however, I think it may be best to make one point. Chaos theory itself is a highly mathematical field of non-linear differential and difference equations. The problem is to model correctly the pieces of reality in which one is interested. A second form of chaos has been invented by those who ignore the mathematics. This latter form is ideologically based. The former is entirely mathematically based and, in one sense a product of the computer, for it is a computer-enabled mathematics of the eye.

THE CONCEPTS OF CHAOS THEORY

Chaos theory arrived at a time when physics was reaching a point where normal science had lost the ability to handle new and important phenomena. Systems were not able to be modeled and explanations were lacking. Linear mathematics and statistical techniques were proving less useful in resolving problems. Some have even argued (Yorke, quoted in Gleick, 1987:68) that the problem was that physicists had been so used to explaining order that they dismissed disorder as an aberration when it was order that tended to be the aberration. Thus, researchers began to run into more and more disorder (nonlinear systems). Into this picture entered chaos theory, with the discovery of patterns in previously random data. Rather than being considered a new paradigm for physics,[4] however, chaos theory came to be seen as a way to "rescue" normal science. By elaborating on the new models, physicists developed new equations for nonlinear systems. Even more precisely, new methods of mapping relationships over time were developed and these enabled researchers to *see* relationships for the first time in systems that appeared to be random.[5]

The Origins of Chaos Theory

Most treatments of the history of chaos theory begin with the work of Edward Lorenz (1963). Lorenz was attempting to find a reasonable time-series model for weather and was charting the output on a computer. In using a three-equation model (a relatively simple one), he made an accidental discovery: very small beginning values in variables could produce vast differences in long-range weather models. Put another way, very small degrees of change made dramatic differences in weather time series. He called this effect an "extreme sensitivity to initial conditions" (see Figure 6-1). His classic example was that "a butterfly flapping its wings in China could affect the pattern of future weather in the United States."

The upshot of this is that the small, random effects found in nature are myriad. Forecasting weather is a reasonably accurate process for a day or two but then loses accuracy rapidly until the deterioration beyond six or seven days makes the forecast worthless. This sensitive dependence on initial conditions is now called the "butterfly effect."

The Butterfly Attractor

A second contribution by Lorenz was his continued search for something more than randomness in the weather data. After all, there were some patterns to weather, and it was obvious that weather was not fully random (e.g., it does not snow in the summer). Thus, he began looking at systems that never quite reached a steady state: aperiodic systems. He finally found a variable (heating by the sun) and a simple equation that handled the repetition in weather models. The conclusion was that the butterfly effect was necessary to keep weather from ultimately locking into a stable pattern and repeating itself over and over. Lorenz then began playing with other nonlinear systems of three or more differential equations. Another classic of chaos theory appeared: the Lorenz attractor, later called the "butterfly attractor" for its shape.

The Lorenz attractor modeled the working of a waterwheel. It had long been known that a waterwheel (think of a waterwheel powering a grindstone at a mill) would unpredictably reverse itself when water flowed over it too fast. The faster the wheel spins, the less time the "buckets"coming down have to fill up and the more likely it is that the buckets on the way up have water remaining them. Thus the equilibrium of the wheel is affected. Over a long period of time, the spin of the wheel will reverse itself many times. When the behavior of the Lorenz attractor is mapped in three-dimensional space over time, it bears a strong resemblance to butterfly wings (see Figure 6-2).

The significance is that such an attractor never repeats itself; no point or pattern ever reoccurs. Yet, the behavior of the entire *system* stayed with the bounds of the butterfly shape, i.e., order out of disorder. Systems that resemble such a shape include electrical dynamos and the earth's magnetic field.

The Horseshoe and Phase Space

The second discovery was that stability and chaos were two different things. After all, the Lorenz attractor was stable—no matter what one did to interfere with it, the butterfly pattern always returned. A mathematician and topologist, Stephen Smale, began examining nonlinear oscillators (1967). The range of possibilities in the oscillation is referred to as the entire phase space, any specific time in the oscillation is a point in phase space. Smale found at least one oscillating shape that changed patterns and left unpredictable points when he stretched and bent it into the shape of a horseshoe (and repeated that interference indefinitely). The real-life analogy to Smale's horseshoe is a taffy-pulling machine. Overall, his work resulted in the recognition of different patterns in phase space (see Figure 6-3). Phase space is merely the bounded graphical representation of the pattern, over time, of a system. Thus, in the butterfly attractor the representation of the wings correspond to phase space.

Bifurcations

Robert May (1976; and with Oster, 1976), a biologist working on population growth, using a simple equation. He discovered that by manipulating one term of the equation, the "boom" and "burst" cycles so prevalent among wildlife, the results ranged from extinction to chaotic complexity. When the parameter was low, growth settled into a stable state; when the parameter was high, growth was unpredictable. May's insight was to plot the results (see Figure 6-4). What he found when the value of the parameter reached 3.0 was bifurcation, a splitting of the data in two with each direction oscillating every year. When the parameter value was 4.0, the data bifurcated into four oscillations. At certain points, then, the growth rate bifurcated (2, 4, 8, 16, 32 oscillations) and oscillated between the bifurcations. The next step

Figure 6-1. Example of Sensitivity to Initial Conditions.

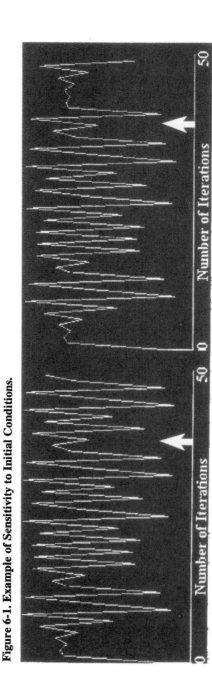

The only difference between the two graphs above is that an initial parameter was changed from 10.0 to 10.0000001. The result is that after 40 iterations the graphs diverge.

Figure 6-2. Lorenz' Butterfly Attractor.

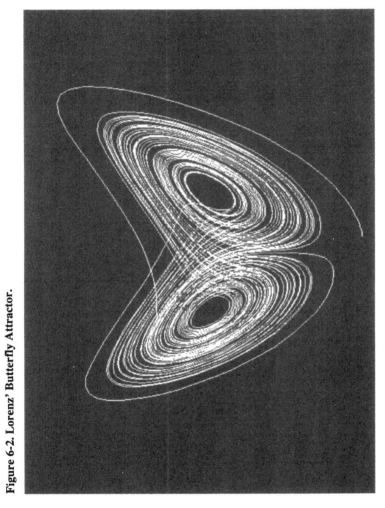

Note the oscillation around the two "eyes" of the wings.

Figure 6-3. Smale's Horseshoe.

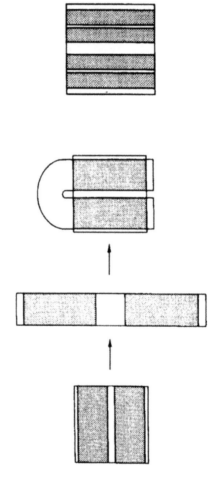

As the figure is stretched and bent, points that originally were close together become randomly far apart.

Source: Illustration by H. Bruce Stewart and J. M. Thompson (1986) *Nonlinear Dynamics and Chaos*. Chichester: Wiley, p. 64.

Figure 6-4. May's Bifurcation Chart.

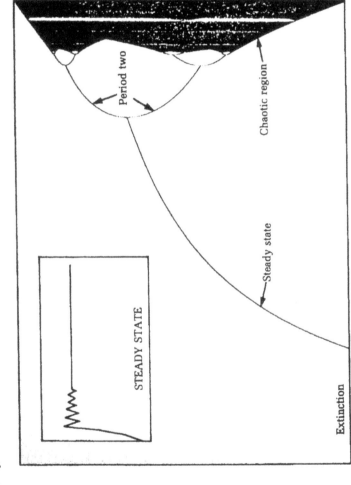

Source: Illustration by James P. Crutchfield and Adolph E. Brotman, from James Gleick (1987) *Chaos: Making a New Science,* New York: Penguin, p. 51.

beyond the highest oscillation point yielded chaos, an unpredictable growth.

Even here, though, an amazing thing happened: in the midst of deep chaos, a window would open in the graph where a periodic, stable pattern returned. This pattern, however, was not a doubling-multiple (i.e., 3 or 7) and immediately bifurcated into deep chaos again. Mathematician James Yorke (Yorke and Li, 1975) was simultaneously working on the same problem and demonstrated the same results for any one-dimensional system hitting what he called "period three" (Mays' 3.0 value for the modified parameter). The same paper used the term "chaos" in the title, and thus chaos "science" and the concept of bifurcations was born.

The Mandelbrot Set and Fractals

Another major concept of chaos theory derived from the work of Benoit Mandelbrot (1977; Berger and Mandelbrot, 1963), a mathematician who dabbled in several other fields. His contribution was that of symmetry of scale. Economists had long assumed (as did scholars in other fields) that small, short-term fluctuations (in prices) had nothing to do with large, long-term changes in a time series. In examining a set of data on cotton prices, it became clear to Mandelbrot that economists were wrong. The problem was that if the small changes were examined at all, they were examined separately from the larger ones. Mandelbrot analyzed them together, and what he found was that the curves of daily price changes exactly matched the curves of monthly price changes. In short there was symmetry of scale, which he applied to other data as well (noise in telephone lines, the rise and fall of rivers, coastlines). From this, Mandelbrot eventually proposed a dimensional geography about irregular shapes with a constant degree of irregularity across scales. He gave this the name of "fractal" geometry. An example of a fractal geometry is in Figure 6-5, which is the Koch curve, or snow-flake. The end result of what are now called Mandelbrot sets is an awareness of self-similarity, of patterns within patterns within patterns as the scale gets smaller and smaller.

Figure 6–5. The Mandelbrot Set.

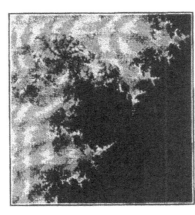

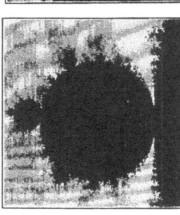

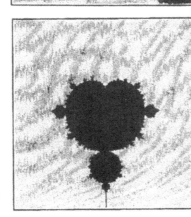

The three graphs above represent a graphed function that is infinitely deep and semi-self-similar. The middle graph is a zoomed-in view of the bump on the top of the leftmost graph. The rightmost graph is a zoomed-in view of one of the small bumps on the middle graph, which, in turn, is a bump on the first graph. Note the repetitive similarity in the detail.

Strange Attractors

The final historical concept I wish to introduce is the notion of *strange attractors*. This is not the end of chaos theory; far from it, there is much more to know. But strange attractors and their basins present the major ideas that were responsible for the development of complex adaptive system theories, where a substantial number of chaos theorists now hang their hats. The concept of strange attractors, and their discovery, is credited to David Ruelle (1980; Ruelle and Takens, 1971), a mathematical physicist. In studying fluid turbulence, a topic considered sophomoric in the physics of the time, he conceived of an attractor in phase space. This wasn't the first examination of an attractor, physicists had already analyzed a point attractor (steady state) and a limit attractor (repeated cycles). Ruelle's contribution is that he added fractals (although the word had not yet been invented) to the picture and thus conceived of an attractor, the "strange" attractor, that would produce every kind of rhythm within phase space. And a picture of one had already been produced—the Lorenz butterfly.

The remaining concept, to be worked out by several chaos theorists was that of a *basin* or point (it can even be a generalized region) in phase space which contained the attractor and around which the regularity of a system settled. Obviously, one critical ingredient in the search for any system is that of finding its basin(s).

The Basis of Chaos Theory: Phase Space and Attractors

First, it may be worthwhile to note that chaos theory has mostly been subsumed under the new nomenclature of *complex systems theory*. In describing the basic elements of chaos theory, I will be merging both old and new ideas. Additionally, it should be understood that chaos/complexity theory is a product of the computer age. Without the power to do reiterative calculations by the millions and then map the result (the reason for calling this a mathematics of the eye), there would be no theory.

The two major concepts are phase space and attractors. Together these are used to create a computer-mapped image of a complex system. Time is always an ingredient in chaos theory. One point in time is calculated and stored, other points are similarly treated and, finally, with thousands to millions of points, the dynamics of the systems can be pictured. Thus, chaos theory is a *dynamic* theory. The more orderly a system is, the more likely it can be represented with traditional linear equations. Less orderly systems are likely to have feedback loops and to be nonlinear, thus requiring a chaos mapping technique. The more complex the system, the more difficult it is to find any form of hidden order. This is the point where attractors become useful but, of course, the task is to find them.

There are probably any number of attractors, but they are currently classified into four types (see Figure 6-6): point attractors, limit attractors, torus attractors, and strange attractors.

A point attractor, the first diagram on the left bottom of the figure (the top diagram represents a traditional 2-dimensional graph of the same phenomenon), is one which creates a point of convergence. The traditional example is a pendulum that swings to and fro, continually decreasing its swing, until stopping at exactly the same point every time (velocity of 0, position of 0). The stopping position is the attractor.

A limit attractor (the next diagram to the right) allows infinite variation between two set boundaries—the extremes of the phase space. It is possible to conceive of the limit attractor in the pendulum example as well. Imagine that, instead of being free-swinging, an outside force (say a motor) applies a push to the pendulum. If the push is exactly the same every time, the pendulum's swing becomes fixed, i.e., "limited." However, the motor is not needed every time the pendulum swings because the pendulum will maintain itself within a slightly decreasing swing. The motor needs to push only occasionally and only needs to push when the swing of the pendulum decreases to a specified amount. Thus, the pendulum is free to vary within the limits of maximum swing and a specified minimum swing. Another example of a limit attractor is that of a thermostat. The thermostat only turns a heater or air conditioner on when the temperature rises or falls beyond a prescribed limit. The feature of limit attractors is that they create stable *cycles* and are even referred to by some as cycle attractors.

The torus attractor (second diagram from the right) is the essence of the Mandelbrot set. It is a pattern in phase space that does not repeat itself but has limits on its variation (sort of an infinite irregularity in a finite space), thereby creating self-similarity in scale. A good example of a torus attractor in nature is a cauliflower plant. The individual pieces in the head of the cauliflower are quite irregular, but there are patterns in its shape. Each segment of the cauliflower is similar to the whole. If you break down the segments, you will again find similar shapes, and so on (a cauliflower is limited by nature in how far it can repeat itself—mathematically generated fractals are not). One

Figure 6-6. The Four Types of Attractors.

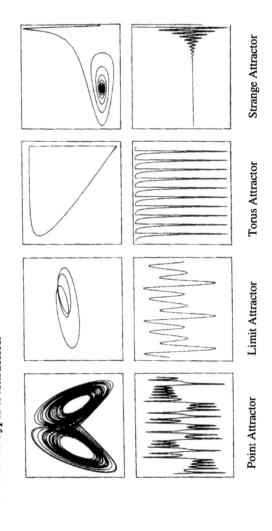

Point Attractor   Limit Attractor   Torus Attractor   Strange Attractor

Source: Illustration by Irving R. Epstein, from James Gleick (1987) *Chaos: Making a New Science*, New York: Penguin, p. 50.

application of fractals is in the creation of graphics on computer screens. Traditionally, graphics are bit-mapped to each pixel on the screen, i.e., instructions are written for each "spot" on the monitor. With fractals, any part of the screen that duplicates another (a blue sky background, for instance) can simply be described once as a fractal and then duplicated as many times as necessary.

The final type is the strange attractor (the rightmost diagram). This attractor is characterized by bifurcations, or splits, in what began as order (a steady state single line). The bifurcations yield multiple basins that, should they continue, ultimately develop into unpredictable points and, as noted previously, redevelop windows with a minimal number of bifurcations and then descend into chaos again. The Lorenz butterfly is the example in the diagram, but the earlier diagram in Figure 6-3 is an example of a more complex strange attractor. Such diverse real world phenomena as measles outbreaks, wildlife populations, protein production, stock markets and the orbits of galaxies have been found to comply with the deterministic chaos "laws" of strange attractors. Mitchell Feigenbaum (1978, 1979) managed to develop those laws in a more universal fashion when he was able to calculate values that resulted in exact points where bifurcation occurs. Moreover, his work showed the relationship between all of the types of attractors. At a Feigenbaum value (as they are now called) of 3.0, a limit attractor will occur, at 3.4495 a torus attractor occurs, and at 3.56 a butterfly attractor occurs. Beyond this point other bifurcations occur at values with increasingly smaller differences and deep chaos will appear.

The Major Features of Chaos Theory

From all this, three major points emerge from chaos/complexity theory.

- *Chaotic systems are deterministic.* Each system has some equation that rules its behavior, no matter how chaotic it appears.
- *Chaotic systems are very sensitive to the initial conditions.* The
  slightest of changes to the starting point can lead to entirely
  different outcomes. Because of this, the systems are relatively
  unpredictable in real life.
- *Chaotic systems appear to be disorderly, even random, but they
  are not.* Truly random systems are not chaotic. Chaotic systems
  have a sense of order and pattern, although it may not be easily
  discernable. Truly orderly systems (those linear systems

predicted by classical scientific methods) are actually the exceptions in the real world; chaos is the common pattern.

The concepts involved in chaos theory seem to apply to human behavior, at least on the surface.

A Few Implications of Chaos Theory

The question now is what can be done with this? There are some intriguing possibilities. First, any chain of events can have a point in which a small change will magnify the results to a threshold of crisis. When translated to behavior, or social reaction, such a possibility tells us that the "major" variables we have been examining in the hopes of explaining criminal behavior may have been off the mark and are simply the variables we notice. Second, the effect of small differences at starting points quickly suggests reasons why our current prediction tools do not do well. We often measure so grossly that small differences are ignored. Third, the same point may demonstrate why individuals who appear to have the same characteristics behave entirely differently. Fourth, self-similarity in scaling suggests that different levels of explanation and analysis may be reconcilable or, at the least, there may be some levels where we find results easier to interpret (e.g., individual vs. structural explanations). Fifth, the recently developed life-course perspective may benefit from chaos theory's dynamic forms of analysis (see Vila [1994:343] on this point). Finally, the implications of nonlinear methodology may force criminologists into other research and analysis paradigms.

In addition to this introductory summary and suggestions, readers should be aware that chaos is a broad field at present. There are those who are at work in subfields (see especially the work of the Santa Fe Institute),[6] and chaos/complexity-oriented research is now spanning virtually all disciplines. Indeed, it is one of those subfields that I now turn to, mainly because of a concern that the breadth of chaos concepts will be difficult to adequately translate to the social sciences. A potentially valuable approach lies in the more limited concept of critical incidents and points (variables) that generate a reaction simply because they are the *final* pieces of a series of effects. A recently elaborated scheme in theoretical physics shows promise as a way to resolve this problem.

A LESSON FROM PHYSICS: SELF-ORGANIZED CRITICALITY THEORY

One of the long-term problems in physics has been to find methods of explaining or modeling very complex systems where standard statistical methods found nothing but random error. Chaos theory offered a broad way to attack this problem, but until recently did not have enough specificity to generate appropriate models. Although there are many applications of chaos/complexity theory now being developed for the social sciences,[7] the problem still arises that there may not be many social phenomena that fit current analytical models. McCleary *et al.* (1996:233–234) argue that the impact of chaos theory in the social sciences has thus far been minimal and that "chaos-type models are not well suited to the problems of modeling economies, societies, and polities." They do suggest that complex adaptive systems may be particularly appropriate for large-scale social phenomena, however.

One form of a potentially suitable complex adaptive system has been formulated by Per Bak, Chao Tang and Kurt Wiesenfeld (1988). They have developed a theory of self-organized criticality to explain behavior in composite systems of millions of interacting elements over a short range of time. Because of its application to complex systems, it should be clear that some version of this theory may be potentially applicable to human behavior.

Origins

The essence of the theory is that "systems naturally evolve to a critical state in which a minor event starts a chain reaction that can affect any number of elements in the system" (Bak and Chen, 1991:46). The chain reactions can be of all sizes, producing anything from minor change to major catastrophes. The size of the event (or variable) itself is of little consequence, the same mechanism is involved with all sizes of effects. Further, Bak and Chen note that "composite systems never reach equilibrium but instead evolve from one metastable state to the next" (Bak and Chen, 1991:46). In short, they postulate that equilibrium is not a normal state, instead favoring change and crisis. Bak and others have continued to develop the approach (see Bak and Paczuski, 1995; Carlson and Swindle, 1995), but its rudimentary form is sufficient for this discussion.

The Paradigm

The paradigm for the theory is a sandpile. As grains of sand are dropped on the same location, the initial resting point of each grain is random. With continued dropping of grains, a familiar shape, a sandpile, begins to develop. As the grains collect, the sandpile grows, until the slope of the sandpile becomes too steep and the grains slide down. With more grains added, the slope becomes steeper yet and the slides become more numerous and larger. When the pile reaches the point where the dropped grains remaining on the pile are, on average, equal to the dropped grains that fall off the pile, a critical state has been reached. Grains added after this point can cause a slide of any size, including a catastrophic one; however, most of the added grains will not cause a slide of any type. Generally, the pile will maintain a critical state by evolving from one critical state to the next. Or, the sandpile will go from a peaked shape to a flatter shape and back again, repeating that general behavior until the system itself is disturbed. During this time, of course, the sandpile grows ever larger.

Predicting Global Features

The theory of self-organized criticality is noteworthy because it does not depend on micro-mechanisms in order to analyze and predict the global features of systems. This means that individual idiosyncrasies and features are not particularly useful in understanding the larger features of the system. The real analytical value lies in the repetition of the shape itself and the point of crisis. Thus, regardless of the individual behavior of components, the overall structure of the system remains the same. This is not to say that smaller portions of the system may not suggest the features of the whole. In fact, evidence indicates that subsets of components will generate the same mechanics as the whole, except for catastrophic reactions, which are dependent on entire structures (Bak and Chen, 1991).

Flicker Noise and Weak Chaos

Two other concepts are also important parts of self-organized criticality theory: flicker noise and weak chaos. *Flicker noise* is defined as a variance in reactions over time, in such a fashion that the reactions vary both in size and duration. Such noise is commonly interpreted by physicists as the effect of past events on current events. In nature, flicker noise appears rather ubiquitous. The theory suggests that this noise is produced when a dynamic system reaches a critical state. In short, just when a system is theoretically most interesting, noise increases. *Weak chaos* refers to unpredictability in the short range only, while fully chaotic systems are simply unpredictable in any time scale. When in their critical state, dynamic systems emit reactions as flicker noise, which is chaotic in the short term but, on average, predictable in the long term. In other words, individual events are relatively random while their aggregate products can be systematic.

The Research Evidence

Evidence in support of self-organized criticality theory has been found in research on earthquakes (Bak and Tang, 1989; Sornette and Sornette, 1989), forest fires (Bak, Chen, and Tang, 1990), rivers (Yam, 1994), economic markets (Bak and Chen, 1991), geographic regions (Stern, 1992) and psychology (Barton, 1994). It seems that the theory may indeed have reasonable application among dynamic systems with many interactive components and may fare well in explaining otherwise chaotic appearances. In spite of its potential for explaining socially complex events, it does not appear that the approach has yet been applied in social research or theory although the larger field of chaos theory has been certainly been used.

NOTES

1. Sections of this chapter first appeared as an article in *Social Pathology* (Williams, 1996).

2. The term "chaos" has different meaning than "random." Randomness connotes full unpredictability; chaos signifies a form of structure *and* unpredictability. At the static level of a point (a datum), unpredictability exists in chaos. At the dynamic level of a system, however, there are patterns and structures to be found. Thus, the use of the word chaos in this book implies, at a minimum, a semi-structured, dynamic system with unpredictable individual points.

3. Stochastic statistics assume random error distributions. Thus, all such techniques compare and partition variance into systematic forms and random forms. If random variance has more weight (the process for determining the amount of weight varies by technique), the result is interpreted as "no relationship." All random variance is considered to be error.

4. There are, indeed, some who perceive chaos theory as the long-awaited mainstay of a new paradigm—anti-positivism. One good treatment of the difference between chaos-as-theory and chaos-as-metaphor (their terms) can be found in Richard McCleary, Richard Crepeau, and Kathleen Dallaire's (1996) recent article in *Social Pathology*.

5. For introductions to chaos and complexity theory see any of the following (the level of mathematics needed for understanding varies, however): Abraham and Shaw, 1992; Eubank and Farmer, 1990; Gleick, 1987; Hilborn, 1994; Holland, 1992, 1995; Murray, 1995; Sandefur, 1993.

6. A summary of their mission and list of publications is available on the World Wide Web at http://www.santafe.edu.

7. Jeff Walker (1996) recently presented a paper at the annual meeting of the Academy of Criminal Justice Sciences that applied strange attractors (specifically, bifurcation systems) to neighborhood disorganization and crime. The paper is quite intriguing but awaits the analytical technique to carry the ideas into reality.

REFERENCES

Abraham, Ralph, and Robert Shaw (1992). *Dynamics: The Geometry of Behavior*. Reading, MA: Addison-Wesley.

Akers, Ronald L. (1985). *Deviant Behavior: A Social Learning Approach*, 3rd ed. Belmont, CA: Wadsworth.

Anderson, Nels (1923). *The Hobo*. Chicago, IL: University of Chicago Press.

Bak, Per, and Kan Chen (1991). Self-organized criticality. *Scientific American* 264(1): 46–53.

Bak, Per, Kan Chen, and Chao Tang (1990). A forest-fire model and some thoughts on turbulence. *Physics Letters* 147(5–6): 297–300.

Bak, Per, and Maya Paczuski (1995). Complexity, contingency, and criticality. *Proceedings of the National Academy of Sciences of the United States of America* 92 (Jul 18): 6689–6696.

Bak, Per, and Chao Tang (1989). Earthquakes as a self-organized critical phenomenon. *Journal of Geophysical Research* 94(B11): 15635–15637.

Bak, Per, Chao Tang, and Kurt Wiesenfeld (1988). Self-organized criticality. *Physical Review A* 38(1): 364–374.

Barton, Scott (1994). Chaos, self-organization and psychology. *American Psychologist* 49: 5–14.

Berger, J.M., and Benoit Mandelbrot (1963). A new model for the clustering of errors on telephone circuits. *IBM Journal of Research and Development* 7: 224–236.

Bernard, Thomas J. (1987). Testing structural strain theories. *Journal of Research in Crime and Delinquency* 24: 262–280.

Carlson, J.M., and G.H. Swindle (1995). Self-organized criticality: Sandpiles, singularities, and scaling. *Proceedings of the National Academy of Sciences of the United States of America* 92(Jul 18): 6712–6719.

Eubank, Steven, and Doyne Farmer (1990). An introduction to chaos and prediction. In Erica Jen (ed.) *Lectures in Complex Systems: Santa Fe Institute Studies in the Sciences of Complexity, Lecture Vol. 2*. Redwood City, CA: Addison-Wesley.

Feigenbaum, Mitchell (1978). Quantitative universality for a class of nonlinear transformations. *Journal of Statistical Physics* 19: 25–52.

Feigenbaum, Mitchell (1979).The universal metric properties of nonlinear transformations. *Journal of Statistical Physics* 21: 669–706.

Ferrell, Jeff (1993). *Crimes of Style: Urban Graffiti and the Politics of Criminality*. New York, NY: Garland.

Gleick, James (1987). *Chaos: Making a New Science*. New York, NY: Penguin.

Gottfredson, Michael, and Travis Hirschi (1990). *A General Theory of Crime*. Stanford, CA: Stanford University Press.

Hilborn, Robert C. (1994). *Chaos and Nonlinear Dynamics: An Introduction for Scientists and Engineers*. New York, NY: Oxford University Press.

Holland, John (1992). Complex adaptive systems. *Daedlus* 121(1): 17–30.

Holland, John (1995). *Hidden Order: How Adaptation Builds Complexity*. Reading, MA: Addison-Wesley.

Katz, Jack (1988). *Seductions of Crime: Moral and Sensual Attractions in Doing Evil*. New York, NY: Basic Books.

Lorenz, Edward (1963). Deterministic periodic flow. *Journal of the Atmospheric Sciences* 20: 130–141.

Mandelbrot, Benoit (1977). *The Fractal Geometry of Nature*. New York, NY: Freeman.

Matza, David (1964). *Delinquency and Drift*. New York, NY: Wiley.

May, Robert (1976). Simple mathematical models with very complicated dynamics. *Nature* 261: 459–467.

May, Robert, and George F. Oster (1976). Bifurcations and dynamic complexity in simple ecological models. *The American Naturalist* 110: 573–599.

McCleary, Richard, Richard Crepeau, and Kathleen Dallaire (1996). Chaos from disorder: A consumer's guide to the recent literature. *Social Pathology* 2: 230–241.

Milovanovic, Dragan (1994). The decentered subject in law: Contributions of topology, psychoanalytic semiotics and chaos theory. *Studies in Psychoanalytic Theory* 3: 93–127.

Milovanovic, Dragan (1996). Postmodern criminology: Mapping the terrain. *Justice Quarterly* 13: 567–610.

Milovanovic, Dragan (ed.) (1997a). *Chaos, Criminology, and Social Justice: The New Orderly (Dis)Order.* Westport, CT: Praeger.

Milovanovic, Dragan (1997b). *Postmodern Criminology.* New York, NY: Garland.

Murray, James D. (1995). Nonlinear dynamics and chaos. Pp. 419–469 in John M. Gottman (ed.) *The Analysis of Change.* Hillsdale, NJ: Lawrence Erlbaum Associates.

Pepinsky, Harold E. (1991). *The Geometry of Violence and Democracy.* Bloomington, IN: Indiana University Press.

Ruelle, David (1980). Strange attractors. *Mathematical Intelligencer* 2: 126–137.

Ruelle, David (1991). *Chance and Chaos.* Princeton, NJ: Princeton University Press.

Ruelle, David, and Floris Takens (1971). On the nature of turbulence. *Communications in Mathematical Physics* 10: 167–192.

Sampson, Robert J., and John H. Laub (1993). *Crime in the Making: Pathways and Turning Points Through Life.* Cambridge, MA: Harvard University Press.

Sandefur, James T. (1993). *Discrete Dynamical Modeling.* New York, NY: Oxford University Press.

Shaw, Clifford R. (1930). *The Jackroller.* Chicago, IL: University of Chicago Press.

Smale, Stephen (1967). Differentiable dynamical systems. *Bulletin of the American Mathematical Society* 1967: 747–817.

Sornette, Anne and Didier (1989). Self-organized criticality and earthquakes. *Europhysics Letters* 9(3):197–202.

Stern, David I. (1992). Do regions exist? Implications of synergetics for regional geography. *Environment and Planning* A 24: 1431–1448.

Stewart, H. Bruce, and J.M. Thompson (1986). *Nonlinear Dynamics and Chaos.* Chichester, UK: Wiley.

Sutherland, Edwin (1947). *Principles of Criminology,* 4th ed. Philadelphia, PA: Lippincott.

Vila, Bryan (1994). A general paradigm for understanding criminal behavior: Extending evolutionary ecological theory. *Criminology* 32: 311–359.

Walker, Jeffery T. (1996). Chaos theory and social disorganization: A new paradigm for neighborhood analysis. Paper presented at the annual meeting of the Academy of Criminal Justice Sciences, Las Vegas, NV.

Whitehead, John T. (1986). The criminological imagination: Another view. *Criminal Justice Review* 10: 22–26.

Williams, Frank P., III (1984). The demise of the criminological imagination: A critique of recent criminology. *Justice Quarterly* 1: 91–106.

Williams, Frank P., III (1991). Explaining criminal behavior: A critical incident approach. Paper presented at the annual meeting of the American Society of Criminology, San Francisco, CA.

Williams, Frank P., III (1995). An alternative perspective on criminal behavior: Critical incident metatheory. Paper presented at the annual meeting of the American Society of Criminology, Boston, MA.

Williams, Frank P., III (1996). Constructing criminological sandpiles: New domain assumptions from physics. *Social Pathology* 2: 218–229.

Yam, Philip (1994). Branching out: Rivers suggest a new feature of self-organized criticality. *Scientific American* 271(Nov): 26 passim.

Yorke, James, and Tien-Yien Li (1975). Period three implies chaos. *American Mathematical Monthly* 82: 985–992.

Young, T.R. (1991). Chaos and crime: Non-linear and fractal forms of crime. *Critical Criminologist* 3(2):3–4, 10–11.

Young, T.R. (1997). Challenges: For postmodern criminology. In Dragan Milovanovic (ed.) *Chaos, Criminology and Social Justice: The New Orderly (Dis)Order*. Westport, CT: Praeger.

CHAPTER SEVEN

A Critical-Incident Orienting-Perspective[1]

CRITICALITY AND CRIMINOLOGY

This chapter is devoted to sketching the general outline of the metatheory. It should be obvious that the use of self-organized criticality theory, *per se*, in the social sciences may be more difficult than in the natural sciences. A major problem at the micro-level is that of measuring incremental changes and events *as they amass in the life of an individual*. It is easier to measure and observe macro-level reactions, however, and the theory may have more direct application in that area. Indeed, its specification of short-term events as weakly chaotic suggests that analyses of individual behavior will not be particularly productive, unless studied over the long term as in life histories. The macro-level, aggregate products of the behavior of many individuals are another matter entirely. One would expect patterns to emerge that would contribute to a certain degree of predictability of behavioral rates. However, even here, there is the necessity of using long-term data.

Using Criticality Concepts

Chaos theory in general and self-organized criticality, particularly, has some interesting lessons for criminology. There are already several chaos-based commentaries in the social sciences. An on-line search of one common periodical database turned up 202 articles over the past 8 years.[2] Sociological journals alone have published quite a few articles, and a recent issue of *Justice Quarterly* contained an article by Dragan

Milovanovic (1996) with an explanation of chaos concepts as used in postmodern thought. The last issue of *Social Pathology* in 1996 had two articles on chaos topics. The offshoots of chaos theory, however, have thus far only found a small audience in the social sciences. Self-organized criticality theory, with its potential of explaining highly complex systems has not been used at all in criminology.[3] While the theory may still be rather obscure in the social sciences, perhaps one reason that it has received little attention is the problem of translating the concepts from physics to human behavior.

Even though a direct translation of the theory is probably possible, I believe that the theoretical concepts themselves suggest useful perspective from criminology. As a result, I propose to avoid problems of translation by "borrowing" ideas from self-organized criticality theory and subsequently using them to create a related, but different, perspective for criminology. This approach has other advantages as well. The borrowed ideas need not accurately reflect their physics counterparts, nor is it necessary even that the essence of the original theory be accurately portrayed. To further resolve problems of translation, I propose to use the theoretical concepts, not in their original unit theory form but in a metatheoretical perspective. The metatheory,[4] to be referred to as a *critical-incident* perspective, assumes that much of reality is reflected in various, otherwise random, events and behaviors that, over time, accumulate into recognizable shapes and patterns. Moreover, these shapes and patterns ultimately result in similar processes, like the analogy that dropping grains of sand are at first randomly dispersed but ultimately form a sandpile of the same recognizable shape (which then engages in a process of avalanche and rebuilding).

Criticality Assumptions

How will this perspective differ from existing conceptions of social reality? The answer lies in current assumptions that events and behavior are purposive and structured. A critical-incident perspective views only the aggregate products of behavior as potentially structured and is less concerned with the purposive nature of individual, chaotic events. Indeed, the following criticality assumptions elaborate on this view:

1. Dynamic systems are complex, chaotic, and complicated.
2. The accumulation of factors in a dynamic system results in a situation where a final factor serves merely to initiate a reaction.

3. Short-term reactions appear weakly chaotic.
4. Long-term reactions are predictable from background factors in the dynamic system, particularly so as they are derived from the aggregation of short-term reactions.

The final assumption is perhaps the most critical one for criminology because it assures researchers and theorists that at least some crime-related events are predictable. As long as units of analysis are at a sufficiently large level of aggregation, events should be reasonably ordered and patterned over time. Conversely, these assumptions also suggest that individual behavioral events are not predictable, except insofar as some general patterns may emerge over the life course.

As far-reaching as these assumptions are, however, they do not yet do justice to the reality of human behavior. Thus, to these assumptions I shall add the implications of our earlier discussions of change, nonlinear phenomena, analogous events, and subjectivity. Finally, I wish to emphasize that the comments to follow are *not* meant to present a new theory, rather they are meant to suggest an alternative perspective from which to view reality.

THE METATHEORY

A metatheory, or orienting perspective, broadly based on critical-incident assumptions suggests a different way of viewing reality. The existing approach, on the whole, is based on a composite of assumptions that incorporate linearity, proximate cause, an emphasis on quantitative methodology, and a sociological bias. Critical-incident metatheory rejects the *ascendance* of all of these views but incorporates their elements.

Overview

What would a critical-incident perspective provide to an understanding of reality? While this presentation remains exploratory, it is already clear that certain orientations would emerge. A metatheory based on the assumptions above would focus on the "assembly" of variables over time to produce behavior. Moreover, the perspective is not disciplinarily bound. The variables being assembled are biological, social, environmental, psychological, and so forth. This fact alone introduces much more complexity than the sandpile analogy. Pieces of sand, as they are dropped on the same point and accumulate, always create the same shape. Variations exist primarily because the individual pieces of sand are not all the same size. Although Per Bak's original discussion of the sand-pile analogy assumed a controlled setting, even more complexity is introduced in a real-world setting through such outside forces as wind and rain or even irregularities in the base level to which the sand is added. It should be easy to see that the complexity of both human structure and behavioral output creates many magnitudes of greater variation than is possible with a sand-pile. Finally, one might argue that, rather than developing the equivalent of a sand-pile's one recognizable shape, humans develop various shapes, and their behavioral output yields a myriad of patterns.

Human Complexity

Greater complexity emerges from the "contributions" that are deposited to create a human shape. Because the contributors differ, some, such as the biological ones, are obviously deposited prior to others. As with grains of sand, the size of such contributions will differ, except in much greater potential magnitude. In fact, I am not positive that there is a limit on magnitude (think of events and circumstances that create massive trauma for individuals).

Further, it is also possible that the last contribution, instead of adding to the collective, will serve to "take away" some of the earlier contributions. That is, both addition and subtraction are possible. For instance, our common experiences suggest that there are things we do to reduce anxiety and stress in our lives (actually, an entire psychological industry has grown up around such an assumption). Thus, contributions cannot be assumed to always be additive.

There is also no reason to expect that linearity is required, particularly when the evidence produced by chaos researchers points to interaction and feedback as a potentially more common phenomenon than linearity. Thus, interaction is a known real-world phenomenon. If variables interact with other variables in the "pile," then multiplication of their effect is possible as well. In effect, I am saying that a stressful day, for example, does not necessarily happen incrementally. Some event or circumstance creates a degree of stress, and the next event may serve to magnify it.

Finally, it would seem that the variables or contributions to the pile do not need to be present in any particular order, all that is necessary is that the pile begins to assume a particular "shape." We do not, for example, require each member of a community or subculture to have identical experiences at identical times for them to be shaped similarly by the community/subculture. On the level of the aggregate (the subculture itself), theorists tend not to even ask "when" events occurred to develop the subculture and the actual sequence may not be critically important either. It is enough that collective and identifiable shapes develop. Indeed, it is these collective shapes that social scientists have tended to interpret as structural factors.

The Life-Shape

All in all, these accumulated variables ultimately reach a point where something (a behavior) is waiting to happen. The next variable, perhaps even one that contributes only a tiny addition to the pile (hereafter called the "life-shape" to combine the concepts of both pile and shape), may be enough to make the behavior occur, or it may occur only with several more additions (or interactions).[5]

To this point, the propensity for action is similar to the sandpile (except for the introduction of interaction). However, just as the complexity of adding to the life-shape is greater for humans, so too is there is reason to expect that the life-shape is more variable than a sand-pile. Thus, with a certain degree of variability in shape, humans may be expected to vary in the probability of engaging in an act, even though the stage may be set and ready for action. The "act" may even be one of several analogous acts contained in a behavioral set. Later, I shall argue that it is these behavioral sets that we need to explain, not the specific behaviors (which may be chosen somewhat randomly).

Individual Behavior as a Random Function

This latter point is clearly a "glitch" from the perspective of normal science, which tends to view phenomena as either predictable or random. Once a behavior is waiting to happen (what the perspective views as a critical slope or point), the effect of adding a new variable does not assure that the behavior will occur. There may be nonlinear feedback, and the result is that of subtraction. Even if the effect is an addition to the life-shape, a reaction is not necessarily forthcoming. This is because the complexity involved in movement of the slope (emission of a behavior) can generate a weakly random function. Thus, even at the *critical* point, behavior is not predictable.

Nevertheless, over a large number of critical points, one can indeed establish probabilities that some behavior will occur. These probabilities are based on longer-term events and generate identifiable patterns, although not perfect ones. In the terms of chaos theory, the patterns of behavior are generated by attractors, but the individual points (specific behaviors) may be oscillating unpredictably around any of the attractors.

Patterns and Classes of Behavior

Attempting to predict what *form* of behavior, rather than a specific behavior, will occur may be the more strategic problem. From the perspective of a critical point, all that is immediately required is that the stress of the point be relieved (or the slope be diminished). Because the metatheory expects a range of "small to large" behaviors (as in the different size sand-slides in the sand-pile), any behavior will relieve the stress. This does not mean, however, that any behavior or any class of behaviors will suffice. A particular shape should require at least the emission of one of a certain *class* of behaviors (e.g., petty theft, vandalism, malicious mischief, or disorderly conduct). For this reason it should be possible to classify a group of similar behaviors (e.g., stress-related behaviors, excitement-seeking behaviors) and predict the emergence of one of the members of that group. Such a form of behavioral prediction may yield more benefits than the specificity we currently try to attain.

Building and Releasing Stress

Adding more complexity to the mix, we have already noted that even at the critical point a behavior may not be emitted because that function is weakly random. If the critical point randomly remains for an extreme period of time, it becomes supercritical. Under these conditions, the addition of each new variable is more and more likely to produce behavior. Such supercritical stress-relieving behavior is more likely to be seen as spontaneous and potentially more harmful behavior.

For instance, instead of initiating a verbal argument, an individual may immediately escalate to an aggravated assault. This may explain Katz' (1988) robbers "bursting" out in an unpredictable (to the victim) pattern of violence-threatening behavior rather than engaging in verbal jousting.

Once supercritical shapes are recognizable, the perspective may be able to point to "superstressed" groups or individuals with a narrower range of probable behaviors. Human ecology assumes such restrictions in available options when there are stressed populations, why not with smaller groups and individuals?[6]

When stress is relieved, the assembly of variables begins again. If only addition takes place, things will build toward the critical point once more. As one might suspect, the life-shape is not required to start all over again, any more than a sandpile must totally rebuild after an avalanche. Because of this, where there are segments of society in which social, environmental, and biological variables routinely build toward critical points, behaviors are aggregately repetitive. Put another way, once shapes develop it may be difficult to discontinue them— there will remain a strong tendency for the base to rebuild. That which was there before is likely to create the same pattern of behavior just as an attractor keeps oscillations in phase space limited. A person who has emitted a certain form of behavior may be more likely to re-emit that form (what David Matza referred to as the "preparation" component of the will when in drift).

If classes of behavior result from certain shapes, the structural conditions emerge for a continuation of those behaviors, perhaps explaining why some behaviors are so difficult to change. Then, of course, there is a question whether certain shapes are more resilient than others and, if so, why? Chaos research suggests that attractors serve to muffle perturbations and return a dynamic system to the previous state. One possibility is that a life-shape itself is itself a form of an attractor.

Social Reaction

If this approach makes sense for criminal or deviant behavior, then it also makes sense that another form of behavior, social reaction, is also governed by similar rules. Perhaps critical incidents can be used to explain "crime reporting waves" or the rise and fall of various social problems. For instance, a public build-up of stress can result in an outbreak of reaction equally as well as individual stress can result in a criminal act. The public's reaction to (or perhaps recognition of) various social problems may be viewed as a product of social stress and the social problem merely one of the set of analogous issues. The rise of the crack cocaine menace, drunken drivers, and even the war on crime can all be interpreted as a product of the stress of the times.

More importantly, the behavior of social reaction interacts with criminal behavior to make the scenario quite complex. Not only is a critical incident required to produce a critical point for behavior but public/agency reaction surely affects the form, or class, of potential behavior emissions. That is, there are fads (currently popular reaction sets) of both reaction and behavior within any society at any moment. If critical slopes are present in both, the conjunction of behavior and reaction sets is complex but potentially predictable in its pattern.

SOCIAL REACTION AND THE CRITICAL-INCIDENT PERSPECTIVE

The focus on the individual thus far is not meant to diminish the importance of social reaction. The social world transcends the effects of social characteristics, biological and genetic makeup, and physical environment. Clearly, the presence of reactive elements that define and redefine values and orientations to people is a major part of the development and formation of any critical incident. Any contributing factor should add/subtract more or less to/from the life-shape depending on the way that variable is perceived both generally and specifically. Reaction should then be viewed as both a behavior in its own right and as a contributor to the behavior of others. It also should be understood that legal codes are also a form of reaction, albeit a pre-existing form, affecting the subjective environment of the offender.

Social Reaction as Behavior

The critical-incident perspective assumes that there is no substantive difference between any form of behavior. All that has been said about an individual moving toward a potential criminal behavior applies as well to reactive behavior. Thus, the effect of social reaction, and even the form of reaction itself, demonstrates general patterns among groups of people. That is, just as behavior viewed across time or as output from large groups becomes minimally patterned, so, too, does social reaction. Indeed, sociologists unquestionably view social reaction in such a way.

Reaction may be a bit more predictable than is some specific form of behavior, such as theft. Having said this, it should be made clear that reaction is itself a *class* of behavior, not a specific behavior. It is precisely because of this class status that predictability increases; the same is true of "crime" (not specifically some form of crime, such as aggravated assault).

Perhaps these comments would be more clear if I referred to negative and positive reaction. Negative reaction is one that tends to punish or apply stigma. Positive reaction signals approval and reward. There are obviously two different forms of reaction implied in the terms positive and negative. A negative reaction can be assumed to have different effects on an individual than a positive one. But even these are mere classes of reaction and specific behaviors are not yet suggested. For instance, in reaction to an individual stealing a purse, shall one frown? Or shall one engage in stoning the perpetrator? The strength and type of reaction are, then, implied in the specific behavior of reacting. Yet, it is possible that any number of specific reactions will have the same effect on another's behavior. If so, reaction may be treated as more of a class than a specific and, thus, be more patterned. Nonetheless, if reaction is to be perceived as a specific behavior, it must be weakly chaotic in its emission.

Reaction as a Background and Foreground Factor for Others

The effect of social reaction on any individual is two-fold. First there is the effect of previous reactions to an individual's behavior. In critical-incident terms, previous reaction is part of the events creating the current life-shape. No less than the concrete variables and factors that make up the rest of the background,[7] previous reaction adds or subtracts from one's life-shape and thereby affects the emergence of a critical slope. This form of reaction then operates as part of the background.[8] Current reaction constitutes the second effect, yet it is obviously not isolated from previous reactions. Previous reactions operate as background factors against which potential current reactions are judged and evaluated in the foreground. The foreground effect results in reaction becoming one of the ingredients in the offender's movement toward a critical point.

In the foreground, reaction is present in several criminological concepts. The notion of situation and opportunity suggests that either there are no potential reactors or that circumstances are such that the reaction will be ineffectual. Both of these imply that the potential offender does not have to assess the chances of success in committing a crime, instead they contribute to the overall environment for crime.

Similarly, the concepts of capable guardians and suitable targets assume that offenders make rational assessments of their social reaction environment prior to making the decision to offend. The latter actually brings the concept of victim into play as another contribution to the offender's life-shape and critical slope. All of these, however, are tempered by the subjective perception of the offender.

Subjectivity and Reaction

Subjectivity is an important part of the reaction framework. In viewing the behavior and character of others, a potential reactor makes a subjective decision. This decision is likely based on his/her assessment of the other and the "harm" imputed to the behavior or potential behavior of the other. The greater the imputed behavioral harm and the more negative the assessment of the offender, the greater is the likelihood of reaction. Such a process matches the elements described by Garfinkle (1956) in his comments on successful degradation systems.[9] For instance, Garfinkle noted that those being successfully denounced need to be socially separated from "normal" people. A negative assessment of an offender serves this process. Where the offense itself is concerned, the conception of harm is potentially even more subjective. As Becker (1963) first observed, the behavior need not have even have occurred, the reactor merely need believe that it has. Indeed, the social-reaction perspective (or labeling) has much to say about the subjectivity inherent in assessing the offender and the offense. More comments on subjectivity and behavior follow in Chapter Nine.

CONCLUSION

There are currently several intriguing ideas emerging in criminology and the social sciences generally. Among them are the concepts of predicting analogous behavior, the effects of change over the life course, and the appreciation of subjectivity. Further, both researchers and theorists are showing an increased recognition of complexity, and statistical techniques are now being used that allow modeling of nonlinear relationships. In choosing a chaos-based form for viewing reality, I have attempted to incorporate these elements.

Most importantly, I believe reality can be best explored as a highly complex series of interacting systems. While criminology has explored virtually all of these systems, rarely has there been any concerted effort to incorporate them as a whole. Most often, we act as if only one or two of them exist and attempt explanation on that basis. These areas are motivation (psychological and social preparation, urges and frustrations), physical environment (lack of defenses, target enhancements), ecological systems (neighborhood deterioration, social disorganization), opportunity (lack of capable guardians, availability of suitable targets), ability (physical capability to perform an act), personal controls (parents, peer groups, internalized prohibitions), legal controls (probability of apprehension and punishment), social reaction (probability of reaction to an act), and making of the legal code (lawful prohibition of acts). All of them are part of the whole envisioned by a critical-incident perspective. And, without treating each one specifically, that is what I hope to convey.

At the risk of missing something, I will summarize the perspective as follows. Behavior of any type is a product of the nonlinear accumulation of multiple systems of factors and variables.[10] The effect of these is then indirectly funneled through the individual's subjective reaction to their presence. A similarly complex system of reaction behavior intrudes into the process, both in a subjective and objective fashion. In this way, a critical-incident perspective tells us that unit theories should encompass object behavior, outside influences on variables creating that behavior, and organizational/reactive elements that serve to define the behavior.

The next chapter continues the presentation of the perspective by adding specifics and details to the concepts discussed thus far.

NOTES

1. This is an elaborated and modified version of materials that originally appeared in *Social Pathology* (Williams, 1996).

2. The database was the Wilson Social Science Index with entries from 1988 to present.

3. At least one other criminologist is now playing with the concepts. After I contributed an early version of this chapter to an internet theory class taught by Jeff Walker at the University of Arkansas–Little Rock, Professor Walker has been working with the general approach.

4. By the term "metatheory" I refer to an orienting perspective. Rather than propose statements about the way in which specific phenomena are related, which is the task of unit theory, a metatheory proposes a way of looking at the world, a way of interpreting and making sense of reality.

5. I wish to make clear that the concept of a "life-shape" is not tied to individuals. It exists in all scales of phenomena. I have used the term life-shape simply because much of the discussion is at the individual level. A group, a society, and a culture all have a life-shape created by their accumulation of factors and events over time.

6. The reality here is that of scales in chaos theory. There is no implicit reason why self-similarities at various scales cannot be translated to behavior at population, group, and individual levels.

7. Jack Katz (1988) also used the terms background and foreground. By background I refer to the composite of variables and factors that have accumulated in the past and are derived from relatively permanent systems. Foreground factors and variables, on the other hand, are those that have recently accumulated or exist in the contemporaneous situation. The latter are likely to be quite transient; the former are usually enduring and intrinsic.

8. There are obvious social-learning implications to these statements. The effect is somewhat like the traditional learning statement that "behavior is a function of past and present consequences."

9. See also John Braithwaite and Stephen Mugford's recent article (1994) on successful reintegration ceremonies.

10. Here I mean to include *internal* and *external* factors and variables. Thus this component incorporates the physical, social, and psychological makeup of the individual and the environmental situation in which the individual finds himself or herself.

REFERENCES

Becker, Howard S. (1963). *Outsiders: Studies in the Sociology of Deviance.* New York, NY: The Free Press.

Braithwaite, John, and Stephen Mugford (1994). Conditions of successful reintegration ceremonies: Dealing with juvenile offenders. *British Journal of Criminology* 34: 139–171.

Garfinkle, Harold (1956). Conditions of successful degradation ceremonies. *American Journal of Sociology* 61: 420–424.

Katz, Jack (1988). *Seductions of Crime: Moral and Sensual Attractions in Doing Evil.* New York, NY: Basic Books.

Matza, David (1964). *Delinquency and Drift.* New York, NY: Wiley.

Milovanovic, Dragan (1996). Postmodern criminology: Mapping the terrain. *Justice Quarterly* 13: 567–610.

Williams, Frank P., III (1996). Constructing criminological sandpiles: New domain assumptions from physics. *Social Pathology* 2: 218–229.

CHAPTER EIGHT

Specific Features of the Perspective

Even at this rudimentary stage of development, there are some very specific implications and features of a critical-incident perspective that will be worth addressing. Indeed, it is possible to make certain statements about what is worth observation and how one might interpret those observations.

MACRO-LEVEL FEATURES

The Accumulation of Variables

The perspective suggests that a large number of variables and factors are responsible for behavior or choices to behave in certain ways. Indeed, this is one of the ingredients that makes the perspective valuable for examining human reality. The variables and factors accumulate during the course of an individual's life, in various "sizes" and "weights." This accumulation creates the life-shape of any individual. At any point prior to a behavior, a culminating variable may be observed. Current metatheory requires an examination of that variable with the assumption that the culminating variable (the one temporally proximate) has an important causal effect. The critical-incident perspective views that variable as no more important in a causal sense than any other variable in the accumulated set. Nor are these accumulated variables required to be patterned in any ordinary, linear sense, although there will be some general precedence.[1] This means that there is no necessary sequence nor logic in the order of occurrence; thus, the presence and sequence of variables will appear to be random. To the extent that *some* ordinary, linear patterns may appear in large samples, any correlation between those patterns and the behavior of interest will probably be small. Critical-incident metatheory suggests that non-linear patterns can be found in behavior over extended periods of time. Those patterns, however, will not be temporally consistent.

Patterns

Because the order of occurrence is not critical does not mean that patterns are not to be expected; some obvious patterns will, in fact, exist among the variables. These patterns, however, will follow the paradigm of weak chaos. That is, they can only be recognized as patterns in the aggregate and then only if sequence is not required. It is these patterns that are found when observing subcultural groups. The rationale for this has to do with the way in which members of a group experience a common environment and background. This means that such patterns can be recognized if order is defined as an aggregate of variables. Moreover, the effect of the aggregate should be contingent on total weight rather than the presence of any singular variable. In short, the more important concept may be what the variables collectively *become* rather than the order in which they accumulated or even the presence of a particular variable in the set. Thus, it should be evident that patterns in group behaviors over time are easier to find, simply because it is likely that individualistic variables are difficult to see. The evidence sociologists look at (and for) is essentially what the individualistic variables have become in groups of people.

CONTRIBUTING FACTORS IN THE LIFE-SHAPE

While the life-shape was discussed in the previous chapter, there are several more concepts that need to be introduced. Some of these concepts are critical to an understanding of the critical-incident perspective and are not simply some "extra" features of the model. These are addressed below.

Weight

The concept of weight is one of the essential elements of the perspective. The presence of a variable is less important than the weight of variables required to produce a behavior or a behavioral choice. Weight suggests that a critical point may be reached by the addition of *any* variable that results in the cumulative achievement of a critical point. Thus, the variable may be conceived of as a "large" variable (childhood socialization, personality type) or a "small" variable (loss of a button, a rainy day). The analogy here is found in the phrase "the straw that breaks the camel's back." A straw, of course, cannot break a camel's back. Once a sufficient amount of weight is placed on the camel, though, a tiny amount of extra weight (the straw) may be all that is needed to reach the critical breaking point.

In one sense, the variable that produces the critical point is no more important than any other variable in the totality. The final variable is just that, the *final* variable. The temporal sequence where different variables are added could easily be switched. As opposed to traditional models where variables are additive, the concept of weight does not imply that there is a steadily accumulating, linear function represented in the summing of variables. To the contrary, the assumption is that the addition of a new variable can be expected to commonly produce an interactive effect such that the overall weight may be increased (or decreased) by a greater amount than the variable itself. Finally, weight also implies that, because it is the cumulative effect that is important, no single variable is critical. That is, any variable may be replaced by another.

Structures

The earlier discussion of patterns in life-shapes implied that there may be specific variables and factors that exist, and have effect, as a group. These grouped variables will be termed "structures." These structures can be found among subsets of factors and variables within a larger assemblage, similar to the various self-similar appendages in a Mandelbrot set. Perhaps another way to conceive of structures is as analogous to smaller versions of the larger life-shape. Their effect is that of generating predispositions for the larger shape by virtue of the structure they create by their grouping. For instance, in the sand-pile example, if certain circumstances result in a fusing together of some of the sand particles, the resultant structure is a smoother surface which will predispose the sand-pile toward avalanches rather than smaller events. While not necessarily requiring the presence of *specific* variables, structures do require that *some* variables in a class of variables exist (although in no particular temporal order). Because they are likely to be more patterned than the individual contributions to the life-shape and, because of their internal linkages, they are more likely to be observed.

It is this phenomenon that is often observed and confused with causal mechanisms. Structures do not act causally but their presence may serve to predispose certain choices or behaviors. For instance, some behaviors may be predisposed by stress (or pressures), others by excitement, and others yet by subcultural "values." Stress, excitement, and subcultural values, then, are structures produced by subsets of accumulated variables, neither in any particular order nor in any particular pattern. Other structures may be characterized by the regularity with which some variables appear in the totality. Examples of such variables are certain genetic traits, psychological states, or the sociological staples of social class, race, and gender.

All structures are not the same in their effect on the life-shape. Deep structures are likely to be part of background[2] factors and perhaps interactive in their affect as well, as with geologic deep lines and fissures that affect the strength of an avalanche (behavior subsequent to the critical point). It may be, for example, that Gottfredson and Hirschi's (1990) recent attribution of criminality to improper child rearing is actually a misinterpretation of a deep structure (child rearing) as a causal mechanism. On the other hand, shallow structures are much less intertwined in the life-shape and much more likely to be additive in their effect. The geologic analogy here is to surface cracks that have little capability of changing the strength of an avalanche but help it to begin sooner. An example of a shallow structure might be children's school experiences as they affect relationships with others and, thereby, predispose the child toward accepting definitions of proper behavior from peers rather than parents and authorities. Other human examples of structures might be stress that owes its origin to genetic and psychological anomalies (deep structure) and stress on the job (shallow structure). Finally, I wish to again emphasize that structures are predispositional in effect, not causal, because they no more create a critical point than does any other variable or set of variables.

Critical Variables

If a final variable and the sequence of variables in the life-shape are not indispensable for a critical point, is it possible that common or regular variables are critical ones? For two reasons, I think not. First, those variables commonly found among large groups of people (e.g., poverty, broken homes, age), are probably not *causal* variables within a linear framework. As Sutherland (1947) said fifty years ago in his ninth proposition of differential association, the detection of general variables in criminals is not an explanation of criminality since those same variables exist in those who conform. For example, broken homes are often used as a causal mechanism for delinquency and criminality, yet there are substantial numbers of people who, although having experienced a broken home, remain law-abiding. Similarly, children raised in urban ghettos do not all become delinquents and criminals. In short, the lives of humans, particularly those living in certain environments, may share commonalities; however, these commonalities, or patterns, should not be taken to represent important causal mechanisms, in and of themselves.

Second, it should be clear that a critical-incident perspective does not place importance on the concept of causally required variables. Any number of variables can serve to replace the weight contributed by an assumed causal variable. The only consideration of importance is whether the single variable had an interactive effect. If so, it may take more or less than a one-to-one match in order to facilitate replacement.

General Variables

I do not mean this to convey that the variables that are usually present are unimportant in the production of deviance, for they represent the foundation on which deviance is built. I simply mean here that it will be rare that such variables are the final precipitating event in the production of deviance (i.e., the *critical* event), simply because they *are* so common. Note the earlier statement, however, that a culminating variable is theoretically no more causal than earlier events.

General variables are nonetheless important for the perspective because they more often than not exhibit significant influence on the lives of large groups of people. Such variables are often found in structures (i.e., combine with other variables) and are therefore capable of generating substantial interactive effects when combined with other, less pervasive and often trivial variables. These latter variables are often idiosyncratic and short term in nature (e.g., a singular stressful experience). Even among themselves, general variables can be expected to add or decrease effect in an interactive fashion. For example, contemporary economic conditions play upon a panoply of general variables in ways that are far from linear.

The Critical Point

The term "critical point" has been used in previous commentary but with only a general definition of what it means. More specificity is now appropriate. The critical point is the stage at which any specific behavior is possible and, in the aggregate, predictable. In this sense, a critical point may be analogous to the point at which a bifurcation occurs in a strange attractor. The accumulation of general and idiosyncratic variables ultimately results in a causal mechanism for criminal behavior (or the general class of behavior) through the accumulation of sufficient weight to reach a critical point. As has been already noted, however, the actual attainment of a critical point does not mean that a behavior will immediately occur. The precipitation of behavior at the critical point is a weakly random function. As with the sand-pile analogy, once the critical point is reached behavior is *likely and ready to occur* but not necessarily at that particular point. Indeed, from that point on, the emission of behavior is a random function (although most likely limited to an occurrence in the near future). If behavior is not emitted, the individual normally remains at the critical point.

The exception here is when an event *subtracts* weight, something not possible in the sand-pile analogy. If, for example, a juvenile is at a critical point, imagine the effect of having his mother suddenly appear; weight is lost and the juvenile is no longer at a critical point. For other behaviors, consider the end of a teacher's frustrating day where a critical point has been reached. The teacher notices students skateboarding down the hallway outside the classroom and is about to engage in reactive behavior when the principal phones and compliments the teacher on her work. The critical point loses weight and dissipates as stress is removed, at least for the moment. Because any form of subtraction, simple or interactive, is always possible, it should be clear that the life-shape is always changing weight. Processes operating at the critical point are no exception. A critical-incident perspective is, above all, a *dynamic* approach to understanding reality.

Assuming again that other events occur and *add* to the weight of the life-shape, the same critical point continues with the same random behavioral function. The only added dimension is movement toward a supercritical point with even more implications for the form of emitted behavior. From the point of view of predictability, it should be clear that a critical point for criminal behavior contains possibilities that no behavior, as well as criminal behavior, will be emitted. Thus, in the short term, it is difficult to predict behavior.

The Supercritical Point

Should a critical point be reached, and criminal behavior not occur, three possibilities hold. First, the event may simply be weakly chaotic and other behavior emitted (or no behavior at all). Second, all environmental conditions may not yet be conducive to action, and, at the point they become so, the criminal behavior will follow shortly. Third, a supercritical point may occur. In this instance, accumulation of stress (or the weight of the life-shape) continues beyond the critical point, resulting in a situation where conditions conducive to criminal behavior may finally produce a substantial, spontaneous outburst. In these cases, spontaneous behaviors, particularly violent behaviors, can be viewed as a resolution of supercritical stress points. Interpreted in this manner, it may be that levels of behavioral seriousness or harm are a function of when behavior occurs relative to the critical incident, i.e., the further removed from the onset of the critical incident, the more serious and harmful is the behavior.

Analogous Behavior

If the ability to specify the emission of some specific behavior seems difficult at this point, it gets even worse. Further compounding the lack of short-term predictability, there is also the possibility that the behavior emitted will not be *criminal* behavior. In general, a critical point tends to produce varied forms of similar behavior rather than a specific form (although the varied forms may also remain within a generic type such as property crime). A choice of behavior at the critical point may, for instance, involve any form of aggressive behavior rather than merely criminal behavior. An individual may choose to play handball, assault someone, or go target shooting. This also assumes that the general category of aggression itself is not merely one of a set of analogous excitement-seeking behaviors. If that is the case, then the entire issue becomes even more complex. At this point, the short-term predictability of criminal behavior is now complicated by both the weakly chaotic emission of true criminal behavior and the fact that virtually any form of analogous behavior shares the same weakly chaotic function.

From this brief discussion, it should be clear that the initial choice of a specific behavior is not as systematic as current theories would predict. The major exception to this statement is the general theory proposed by Gottfredson and Hirschi (1990: 42, 91), wherein they acknowledge the lack of specificity involved in criminal behavior and discuss behavioral forms that are equivalent to criminal behavior. This point alone may be a major breakthrough for mainstream theory's understanding of crime as a complex phenomenon. Nonetheless, the simple recognition of analogous behavior is not sufficient. More is needed. In short, an individual reaching the critical point may emit no behavior, any of an analogous set of behaviors, or criminal behavior (which in itself is a loose collection of analogous behaviors). Unfortunately, this does not constitute the end of the complications for prediction.

Flicker Noise

It is, of course, possible that any critical point may occur without the generation of criminal behavior. Under the tenets of the original self-organized criticality theory, a critical slope will emit flicker noise. That is, once a critical point is reached, systems generate weakly chaotic emissions. For our purposes flicker noise represents a weakly chaotic condition under which various forms of individual behavior occur. These behaviors are likely to be of an analogous class but may constitute *any* potential response, thereby tending to obscure (in the short term) even the class of behavior most likely to be emitted. Since a response serves to alleviate the stress of the critical point, it is reasonable to expect the response to be at least of a generic form. That generic form, however, may constitute any stress-relieving behavior. In terms of criminality this means the individual may engage in anything from thrill-seeking to assaultive behavior. Moreover, there is no particular reason to believe the criminal behavior is a unique class of behavior—any stress-relieving response will do. Flicker noise, then, is essentially the set of chaotic, short-term responses.

There may be even worse news for those who are committed to versions of linear, proximate causality—individual subjectivity also plays a part. What may be subjectively reasonable to an individual, given situation and life history, may not be reasonable to an observer. As a result, stress-relieving behavior may not appear to be so when taken out of the individual's subjective context. Thus, all things being equal, predicting the emission of *any* criminal behavior as an individual's reaction at the critical point is difficult. Fortunately for predictability, in the long run an individual's behaviors across many critical points should begin to show patterns. Similarly, critical points are likely to produce criminal (or analogous) behavior patterns across groups of similarly situated people. It is in the individual and short-run cases, though, that the generation of criminal behavior remains exceedingly problematic.

Repetitive Behavior

The picture painted above of individual behavioral responses at the critical point seems to be convincingly chaotic. Under the assumptions of a critical-incident perspective, it appears to be a wonder that *any* action is even mildly likely. Yet we also know that reality is not like this. People who commit an act are more likely to commit that act again (something we know from parole classification research). How then can behavioral choices become partially systematic? Or put another way, how does an attractor develop?

A reasonable answer is based on two factors: the robustness of dynamic systems and the foundation of the life-shape. In the first instance, we already know that most complex, dynamic systems will withstand outside perturbations in their phase space. I.e., they will return to their oscillations around the attractor. The former instance is more a product of the robustness of a life-shape itself. Once the critical point is reached, the likelihood of maintaining a behavior is increased by the continuing presence of factors and variables that served to create the original critical point. That is, because of the existing foundation, a re-emergence of the critical point is likely as long as the previous factors remain. David Matza's (1964) concept of "preparation of the will" is useful here in explaining repetitious behavior. Once emitted, an individual potentially learns a particular response to a particular critical point (see C. Ray Jeffery's (1965) and Ron Akers' (1985) approach to operant learning on this issue). While this does not mean that the individual will *not* choose other alternatives, it does make a repetition in choice more likely. This serves to explain persisting criminality as well as the varied nature of proximate "causes" currently used to explain criminality. It also serves to explain research evidence that most repeat criminals are not likely to engage in a singular behavior but, instead, a variety of criminal acts. That this is so becomes evident when one considers the effect of flicker noise—a class of behaviors is being repeated, not *a* behavior.

Change over Time

The final point to be made concerns the effect of change. Humans appear to change throughout their life course. This fact has been traditionally observed in criminology by the fact that crime is a young person's behavior. Indeed, a standard argument has been that juveniles age out of crime. The corollary is that the elderly have extraordinary low rates of crime. Schur, in his book *Radical Nonintervention* (1973), used the aging phenomenon as the foundation on which he proposed deinstitutionalizing punishment for most delinquencies. More recently Sampson and Laub (1993), in resurrecting and revisiting the Glueck's old data, have presented convincing evidence that change is relatively endemic. Others (Bursik, 1986; Bursik and Webb, 1982; Schuerman and Kobrin, 1986) have examined neighborhoods and determined that the way in which neighborhoods change has been an overlooked factor in ecological studies.

Under critical-incident approach, change is an expected part of reality. Each time a variable or factor is added to the life-shape, change occurs. Indeed, it is this rather simplistic form of change that has been evident in discussions thus far. A greater complexity exists, however, because of the possibility of a new event decreasing (even interactively) the existing collective weight. Such events serve to move the life-shape of an individual back and forth, even on the cusp of a supercritical point. Thus, it is possible that a juvenile at the peak of a life-shape heavily weighted toward criminal behavior will achieve an event (perhaps a meaningful job or the intervention of some close friend) that interactively reduced that weight. Subsequent events may continue the process and create a life-shape more heavily weighted toward conformity. If recent evidence is correct,[3] this is precisely what happens in one form or another.

Multiple Critical Points

Now we arrive at the ultimate point of individual complexity. Because this discussion has focused on the way in which *a* critical point develops and the implications of that single point for behavior, it might seem as if only one critical point develops at any one time. That clearly is not the case; humans are more complex than that. If most behavior can be represented by this perspective, then it follows that there are several critical points in existence at any one time. To borrow a computer-oriented term, humans are "multi-tasking" organisms—they are capable of engaging in more than one behavior simultaneously.

Moreover, stimuli from the environment (internal and external) are not required to affect the individual in a one-by-one fashion. There is no reason that stimuli from real-world conditions would not commonly affect the individual simultaneously. This is another reason why variables that arrive close in time to any behavior of interest should not be perceived as predictors. They may not even be adding to or subtracting from the weight necessary for that particular behavior.[4] Isolating the unique stimuli for a specific behavior is risky. Another possibility is that any one stimulus may have an effect across a range of weights moving toward a critical point.

Having added this final piece of complexity to individual behavior, I want to argue that things are not quite as bad as they seem. Humans do indeed engage in quasi-predictable behavior, especially in those forms that may be classified as rote or repetitive. In those cases I suspect that behavior that originally developed in a typical critical-incident process has been somehow routinized. In reality, these routinized behaviors are the hallmark of normal science. Thus, I do not expect a critical-incident perspective to explain *all* behavior. But, even in these cases, I expect the original development of a routinized behavior to have come from a critical-incident process. Thus, there should be subprocesses operating under the perspective. Those clearly are in need of specification and development.

CONCLUSION

The intent of this chapter was to begin a discussion of the more complex points of a critical-incident metatheory. There are many more details that need to be worked out, but my major purpose was to demonstrate that the cursory theoretical overview presented in the previous chapter is reasonably reflective of reality. I also realize that the complexity of concepts presented in this chapter is difficult to digest and may tend to make one lose sight of the larger orientation. For this reason, I have included a boxed summary at the end of the chapter (Figure 8–1).

At this point, I anticipate that the most likely criticism of the perspective is that all possible actions are possible at the critical point:

Figure 8–1 . A Brief Summary of the Perspective.

1. Chaos approaches emphasize the presence of seemingly random information that under certain dimensions of observation yield rather systematic patterns. Dimensions of observation involve moving up to larger views of phenomena, or moving down to smaller ones. They also involve changing the position of observation and the period of time.

2. A certain offshoot of chaos theory, self-organized criticality theory, suggests that various, otherwise random, events and factors accumulate into recognizable shapes and patterns. Moreover, these ultimately result in similar processes, like the analogy of dropping grains of sand to form a sand-pile.

3. A criminological critical-incident perspective focuses on the "accumulation" of variables over time to produce behavior. The variables being accumulated are biological, social, environmental, and psychological. Some are obviously deposited prior to others, and it is also possible to "take away" some variables. That is, both addition and subtraction are possible, as well as interaction (actually, any function is theoretically possible), and all affect the composite weight of the system.

4. No particular order is required for the accumulating variables. All that is necessary is that the pile begins to assume a particular shape. These accumulated variables ultimately achieve enough weight to reach a critical point where something (a behavior) is waiting to happen. The next variable (perhaps one with a tiny addition to the pile) may be enough to create the behavior.

5. Once a behavior is at the critical point, the effect of adding a new variable does not assure that a particular behavior (such as theft) will occur. This is because the emission of behavior is a weakly random function. Over a large number of critical points or over a large group of individuals, however, behavior becomes patterned and more predictable.

6. Predicting specific behavior is a problem. Any of a similar class of behaviors remains possible, or even a nonclass behavior may occur.

7. If the critical point randomly remains for an extreme period of time, it becomes supercritical. Under these conditions, the addition of each new variable is more and more likely to produce behavior. Such supercritical stress-relieving behavior is more likely to be seen as spontaneous and potentially more harmful behavior.

8. Once a behavior relieves the stress, the "accumulation" of variables begins again. If only accretion takes place, things will build toward the critical point once again. Because of this, where there are segments of society in which social, environmental, and biological variables routinely build toward critical points, behaviors are aggregately repetitive and predictability increases.

9. Criminal behavior itself is only one of a class of behaviors. There are many different forms of behavior that serve to relieve the stress of a critical point. Thus, the task is not to explain criminal behavior per se, but the class of behavior. At aggregated levels, however, rates of crime should increase given accumulations of certain variables for certain groups. Crime rate predictions, then, are more possible.

(continued next page)

(continued)

10. Social reaction is governed by similar rules. Additionally, the behavior of social reaction interacts with criminal behavior to make the scenario quite complex. Not only is a critical incident required to produce a critical point for behavior, but public/agency reaction interacts with and affects the form of emitted behavior.

11. Behavior is also a function of subjective reality, both for the individual acting and those reacting to the response. Therefore, the interpretation of various conditions and stimuli present at any given time affects the nature of the life-shape (the slope) and whether a particular factor is a critical incident.

---

no behavior, the behavior of interest, analogous behavior, and any alternative behavior. This would seem to make the perspective worthless—it predicts everything and nothing. However, it should be true only for the original critical point. Once the life-shape has been built, and if nothing decreases weight, the critical point will occur over and over. When this happens, behavior becomes weakly predictable, if for no other reason than David Matza's (1964) notion of *preparation*. What one has done before is added to the base of future critical points and serves as a potential restriction on future behavior. At any future critical point the former reactions should still remain, but the emission of "any alternative behavior" should be radically reduced to a class of behavior (analogous to limits that create the phase space around a chaos attractor). In short, the point of original behavior still remains problematic but, over time and with repetitions, patterns will begin to emerge within classes of analogous behavior.

I now turn to a discussion of some of the implications of critical-incident metatheory for existing unit theories in criminology.

NOTES

1. It should be obvious that genetic and biological factors are likely to precede most of the psychological and sociological ones. In that sense there is a general order to the deposit of variables and factors making up the life-shape. Within this general order, however, I see no reason to require a certain sequence of occurrence.

2. Jack Katz popularized the use of the terms "background" and "foreground." To prevent confusion, by background I refer to those factors and variables that already exist and are not likely to be removed from the life-shape.

Foreground signifies the contemporaneous events and conditions that are being incorporated into the life-shape or have the potential for incorporation.

3. This is precisely the evidence that Sampson and Laub (1993) found in their data. As the juvenile progressed toward adulthood, it was the gaining of a job, or even marriage and a family, that generated the movement toward greater conformity.

4. I realize this introduces a new possibility here as well. All conditions do not necessarily generate something that affects an organism. It is a truism that organisms do not pay attention to everything in their environment—they cannot afford to or else they would become paralyzed by information. Evolution has probably seen to it that species react to those conditions and stimuli that are critical for survival, or even comfort, thus ignoring benign information. Thus, there must be conditions that are neutral as far as the dynamics of a life-shape are concerned.

REFERENCES

Akers, Ronald L. (1985). *Deviant Behavior: A Social Learning Approach.* 3rd Ed. Belmont, CA: Wadsworth.

Bursik, Robert J., Jr. (1986). Ecological stability and the dynamics of delinquency. Pp. 35–66 in Albert J. Reiss, Jr. and Michael Tonry (eds.) *Communities and Crime. Crime and Justice: A Review of Research.* Vol 8. Chicago, IL: University of Chicago Press.

Bursik, Robert J., Jr., and Jim Webb (1982). Community change and patterns of delinquency. *American Journal of Sociology* 88: 24–42.

Gottfredson, Michael and Travis Hirschi (1990). *A General Theory of Crime.* Stanford, CA: Stanford University Press.

Jeffery, C. Ray (1965). Criminal behavior and learning theory. *Journal of Criminal Law, Criminology and Police Science.* 56: 294–300.

Matza, David (1964). *Delinquency and Drift.* New York, NY: Wiley.

Sampson, Robert J., and John H. Laub (1993). *Crime in the Making: Pathways and Turning Points Through Life.* Cambridge, MA: Harvard University Press.

Schuerman, Leo, and Solomon Kobrin (1986). Community careers in crime. Pp. 67–100 in Albert J. Reiss, Jr., and Michael Tonry (eds.) *Communities and Crime. Crime and Justice: A Review of Research.* Vol. 8. Chicago, IL: University of Chicago Press.

Schur, Edwin (1973). *Radical Nonintervention: Rethinking the Delinquency Problem.* Englewood Cliffs, NJ: Prentice-Hall.

Sutherland, Edwin (1947). *Principles of Criminology*, 4th ed. Philadelphia, PA: Lippincott.

CHAPTER NINE

Implications of a
Critical-Incident Metatheory

INTRODUCTION

The most common approach to constructing criminological theory has typically been to perceive critical explanatory factors as belonging to a single dimension, generally the social, and then to search for the "most important" variables in that dimension. This approach grossly oversimplifies the reality of human interaction and behavior. The complexity of human dynamic systems easily approximates, or exceeds, those of the natural sciences. I have been arguing that it makes more sense to perceive those things we call explanatory factors as the product of years of social interaction, compounded with the effect of biological systems and psychological influences, and mitigated by environmental conditions of the past and present (not to mention social reaction). From this perspective, the most recent, most common, or most visible factor may be at best nothing more than a behavioral preface. At the same time, it may be the preface needed to complete the total causal reaction precipitating the behavior. After elaborating on this perspective in the previous two chapters, I now will explore the implications of a critical-incident approach for criminology.

SOME ISSUES FOR CRIMINOLOGY

A critical-incident metatheory is best seen as an overarching perspective from which to view behavior and methods of analyzing that behavior. From this viewpoint, I propose that the metatheory anticipates the variables and structures emphasized by various existing theories, explains the relatively low correlational evidence for individual-level theories, and clarifies the difficulty of translating structural theories into lower levels of explanation.

General Issues

As a metatheoretical approach, the perspective has several implications for the criminological enterprise. First, the normal pattern of causal logic that seeks parsimonious and proximate[1] causes may be insufficient to capture richly complex phenomena. I am not arguing here that researchers specifically view their variables as "causal," but merely that parsimonious and proximate variables be searched out and used in research. While such variables have served in the past, they now tend to place constraints on understanding. If we know which general concepts are implicated in precipitating behavior, it is time to explore the complexity of the concepts and the relationships. Actually, that is what some contemporary researchers have been doing, and, thus, a critical-incident perspective may assist in defining that complexity.

Second, the inclusion of multi-disciplinary causal variables in theoretical constructions is advisable. If background variables are important in forming the base of a life-shape and are entangled in deep structures as well, it becomes obvious that theories using single discipline concepts are unlikely to explain much of behavior. Criminology needs theories that explain which biological, environmental, and psychological variables are most likely to provide a base. Following that should be theories that explain how such variables interact with social variables to produce a critical point.

Third, if criminal behavior is indeed chaotic (but not random), then structural levels of explanation will be more successful in predicting behavior. However, the form of behavior will tend to be of aggregates or groups over time, i.e., what is commonly known as *rates* of behavior. Individual-level behavior may be potentially predictable but one needs to be looking at the life-course and have an extensive time-series database. Where structural theories exist, it makes sense to spend time exploring and understanding how analogous behaviors affect their predictions. We also need to know how those theories relate to the more individual-level theories of process.

Fourth, dependent variables are better conceptualized as *sets of behavior* rather than unique, independent behaviors to be explained.

The discussion of crime in Chapter Four is a case in point. Crime itself is a vague concept. When combined with a perspective that views any analogous behavior as potentially equivalent (behaviorally, not legally), it becomes obvious that some effort must be spent in determining what sets of analogous behaviors exist. Similarly, what concepts (patterns) serve to create the sets? For instance, is "criminal" behavior part of a set of stress behaviors, or part of a set of excitement behaviors, or both?

And finally, the inclusion of psychological variables suggests that variables affecting an individual may be more properly interpreted from the subjective perspective of the individual (although it is possible that, collectively, subjective interpretations become patterned). Thus criminology needs to know much more about criminal behavior from the perspective of the criminals.

Aggregates and Prediction

One of the concrete contributions of a critical-incident perspective is prediction. It seems obvious that collections of events and factors can be aggregated and used to indicate a group that is "at risk." That is, a group at risk is a group with a collective pattern of events, factors, and variables that assemble in a shape with a critical slope. While the exact prediction of critical slopes is not feasible, it is indeed possible to identify those collective factors (some of which are structures) and variables that commonly act as contributors to certain shapes. It should also be possible to examine groups over time and determine the approximate average onset of critical slopes. If that can be done, higher levels of criminal/deviant behavior can be predicted. This task—the identification of contributors, shapes, and critical slope onset—is perhaps the most important immediate issue facing criminology. It certainly has more promise than most of what criminologists have been doing for the past 50 years.

To assist in prediction, certain regularities seem to appear in the factors and variables involved in forming critical slopes. The most important ingredients for aggregate predictions of the critical slope are probably background factors that serve to maintain the base from which a shape may rebuild. This is due to the building-block effect they provide for most individuals. These background factors are biological, structural, and socialization ones. Both immediate and past experiential variables can be derived from combinations of the background factors.

Further, immediate social reaction variables can probably also be derived from background factors.

One of the problems of contemporary criminology, the similarity of deviants and nondeviants, is actually addressed here. Because the background factors are shared by so many individuals, the commonality among deviants and non-deviants is virtually a given (same basic life-shape). What then separates them? Critical-incident metatheory tells us that the difference is in proximity of the life-shape to the point of generating a critical slope. In other words the problem is not in what people are, the problem is in what they are becoming.

Thus, the tasks for criminology under a critical-incident view of the world are:

- Determine emergent patterns over time in social groups,
- Examine social groups with high rates of deviance (and analogous behavioral sets) over time,
- Identify the general shape (accumulation of variables, events, and conditions) present during periods of high deviance rates,
- Identify the conditions, patterns, and characteristics that indicate the presence of a critical slope, and
- Determine the average onset of critical slopes over time.

I would add the reminder that none of these tasks assume a linear progression to any of the patterns, conditions and characteristics that will distinguish a group-shape[2] with a critical slope.

Time-Order Among General Variables

The presence of general variables and "patterns" may result in evidence anticipated by current theories of behavior, but without either the order or specific variables envisioned by those theories. In fact, the occurrence of theoretically important variables in a substantial number of observed cases can serve to provide support for a theory by providing weak correlations. This is particularly true when the data cannot provide accurate information on the temporal position of the variables as is so often the case in secondary and survey data. Because idiosyncratic variables are often not part of collected data and because general variables are, by implication, generally collected, evidence will spuriously support the theoretical primacy of general variables.

The Lack of Causal Proximity in General Variables

Another major problem of some general variables is that, if widespread enough, they may be equivalent to constants and thus show no relationship to outcomes. That is, large numbers of the population, both deviant and nondeviant, will share the same characteristic, making it impossible to associate the characteristic with behavior. Yet it is possible that many, widely experienced variables lay the necessary foundation upon which other variables appear to build into deviant behavior. For instance, poverty has long been assumed to be a contributor to criminality. Yet, it is not possible to establish poverty as a linear and proximate "cause" of crime because it is too pervasive and not properly linked in time with crime. However, it should be clear that, as a foundation variable, poverty contributes a great deal to the building of other forces that will ultimately yield criminality. This contribution, nonetheless, does not mean that poverty has to be properly time-ordered with these other forces for a critical slope to build. I suspect that something such as poverty (which is a concept, not a unique variable) is tantamount to an interactive deep structure, to use an term introduced earlier.

Using the earlier sand-pile analogy, virtually everyone has a sand-pile made up of similar ingredients; the problem is to determine who has a sand-pile with sides that are too steep. In the critical-incident scheme, a *combination* of variables occurring over time creates a critical point and the resulting behavior. Finally, in a linear world, general variables are unlikely to be among the variables most proximate to any behavior and, therefore, will be commonly assumed to have no effect. Complex non-linearity resolves the foundation/causal proximity property and allows theorists to conceive of important variables that are not, by themselves, causal.

The Use of Behavioral Sets

Theories that deal in structural and aggregate relationships (e.g., strain theories, ecological theories, and routine activities theory) demonstrate the effect of moving up in level of aggregation within a critical-incident perspective. The aggregate patterns predicted by these theories are the results of critical point reactions over multiple trials (individual reactions) over time. Where these theories fail lies in the *type* of reaction predicted. In the case of crime rates, there may be both large and small group increases in rates predicated on the chaotic nature of the sum of the individual reactions. Such individual reactions also will chaotically vary in the type of behavior (of which crime is only one), thus causing the aggregate rates to vary unpredictably in the short term. As Gottfredson and Hirschi (1990: 42, 91) have perceptively acknowledged, there are many forms of behavior that are theoretically equivalent to crime. Whenever criminal outcomes are predicted, equivalent behavioral forms probably should be included as well. If individual reactions are chaotic, a wide variety of behavior may be found at the aggregate level, thus creating problems in predicting and measuring any one, or any specific group, of behavior. Because chaotic behavioral emissions at the critical point may be any suitable (stress-relieving) act, the method of locating patterns is to look for dominant behavioral sets (not a dominant behavior).

One implication of a critical-incident perspective for structural theories, then, is that the variety of expected outcomes must be expanded. As an example, Osgood *et al.* (1996) have recently shown the value of approaching the dependent variable as a concept rather than a single variable. They used a five-wave, national sample of juveniles to determine the relationship between routine activities and deviance instead of focusing on one or two forms of crime. Defining deviance as criminal behavior, heavy alcohol use, use of marijuana and other illicit substances, and dangerous driving, they were able to account for a higher proportion of the variance than if only criminal behavior had been used. In short, by using a variety of outcomes tied to the concept of deviance, they were able to improve prediction of what is otherwise chaotic individual behavior.

Ecological theories can also benefit from chaos-oriented approaches. Theorists and researchers have already recognized that a neighborhood ecological pattern is not static and have begun talking about community change over time (Bursik, 1986; Schuerman and Kobrin, 1988; Walker, 1996). What has not yet been done is to discuss behavioral sets as outcome measures. A sole focus on crime rates can be expected to generate relatively low correlations because crime is only one of the potential collective (neighborhood) reactions. This is particularly important when one adds the dynamic feature of change over time; conditions and reaction sets are likely to be sensitive to the context of changing times.

Theoretical Sets

The critical-incident approach also provides a bridge between theories of motivation (strain theories, cultural deviance theories, subculture theories) and theories of inhibition (control theories, punishment in learning theories). From this perspective, motivators toward deviance are the variables and factors that result in additions to a movement toward a critical slope. That is, they help *add* to (or multiply) the assembly of ingredients that result in a shape conducive to an avalanche (critical incident). Under this conception anomia, or perhaps an excess of criminal definitions, contribute to the overall buildup and weight of an individual's readiness for deviance. Inhibitors for deviance, such as the elements of the social bond, detract from the accumulated factors and reduce the likelihood of a critical slope occurring. Involvement in conventional activities, then, may serve to *subtract* from the general pile of ingredients and reduce deviance readiness.

Certain theories, such as social learning (Akers, 1985), may more closely approximate the processual and individual-level events anticipated by a critical-incident metatheory. A major criticism of social-learning theory has been the problem of reinforcement. If an expected behavior does not occur, then a stimuli expected to act as reinforcement cannot, by definition, be a reinforcer. One plausible explanation has been that the consequences of all past behavior are not known and, therefore, under certain discriminative stimuli, an expected reinforcer will not be so for a particular individual. A critical-incident approach adds the concepts of totality of weight (past consequences and other accumulated factors) and critical point to the typical social-learning scenario. By doing so, an expected reinforcer may be explained as simply a temporally-proximate variable insufficient to create a critical point or that, in this specific situation, the critical point has been reached but, instead of producing an immediate reaction, randomly escalates toward the supercritical point.[3]

Levels of Explanation

Critical-incident metatheory also reaffirms the importance of understanding levels of explanation for theories. As Bernard (1987) has aptly observed, a serious mistake is made in placing the unit of analysis for structural theories at the individual level. Any such attempt destroys the aggregate structure present in the data and can be expected to yield low linear correlations as the product of chaos. Moreover, a prediction of individual *criminal* behavior will fail because criminal behavior is only a chaotically emitted form of the various types of flicker noise. Thus, a structural theory specifying a *particular* form of criminal behavior will be even more difficult to support at the individual level (should such translation even be possible). On the other hand, a theory postulating a general *class* of behavior and keeping its specifications at the aggregate level should prove more predictive.

As an example of this problem, Merton's (1938) anomie theory proposes that deviance increases with the estrangement of cultural goals and socially-approved means to reach those goals. He does not propose this explanation for individuals[4] but refers to rates of deviance among groups. Thus, measuring individual estrangement and attempting to predict deviance will fail because of flicker noise. In a previous piece of research, Marilyn McShane and I (1985) resolved this issue by grouping individuals into levels of social class and calculating their group rates of marijuana use. Assuming that social-class levels provide a measure of the goals-means estrangement, group rates of deviance should increase with the level of social class. That is precisely what we found (actually the relationship was perfect at the ordinal level). Analyzing the same data at the individual level, we found no relationship—flicker noise prevailed. If *multiple* measures of deviance had been available and analyzed as a behavioral set at the group level, we suspect the results would have been even more convincing.

Multiple Measures

It is worth noting that tests of criminological theories tend toward standardizing the independent variables measuring those theories. For instance, tests of differential association theory have frequently used independent variables measuring the number of close friends who commit a form of deviance. Anomie theory and social disorganization theories, at least during the 1950s and 1960s, were standardized on census measures of the proportion of minorities in an area and poverty rates, while arguments revolved around how to rotate the factor analysis using these variables. Hirschi's social control theory has been commonly tested using the same self-report questions that Hirschi himself originally used. By noting these particular theories I do not mean to unfairly point to them—indeed, virtually every theory has been tested in an identical manner. In each case, a concern for making sure the "best and most representative" variables are used has resulted in a uniformity of testing that ignores the desirability of measuring concepts through the use of multiple measures. Triangulation of measures should be more successful in locating the property space of concepts than single measurements (just as triangulation of stars assists in geographical location). By acknowledging the complexity of reality, a critical-incident perspective would encourage multiple measures of concepts, especially those based on variables from multiple disciplines.

DETERMINISM, VOLITION, AND SUBJECTIVITY

A portion of the earlier theoretical critique noted that criminology needed, to paraphrase a classic sociological phrase from George Homans (1964), to bring subjectivity back in. Because the dominant paradigm is objective, such a move will not be an easy one. However, it is possible under a critical-incident perspective to incorporate objectivity and subjectivity as well as determinism and free will.

Determined and Volitional Factors

Background factors of all sorts (biological, environmental, psychological, sociological) are responsible for the general life-shape of the individual. Because of their contributions to the shape, and the likelihood of common experiences, social values, and socio-economic situation among members of similar subcultural environments, aggregate groups (such as members of a subculture) are probably more predictable in their behavior. Put another way, background factors are useful in predicting rates of aggregate behavior (but with the problems discussed earlier under the topic of "general variables"). Thus, a deterministic[5] framework can be expected to mesh better with background factors than with foreground factors.

Foreground factors, on the other hand, are less deterministic. These factors encompass the subjective reality of the actor and are chaotic. Even though objective factors may be available, such as environmental situations or the presence of capable guardians, whether the actor perceives these at the time of decision-making is not an objective fact. This subjective perception of a situation can be defined as *volition* (or free will or rationality) and adds the actor's interpretation of the situation to the equation of behavior. Thus, volition is present at the point any act is performed. An individual brings background factors to a situation and those assist in locating patterns and predicting actions. The foreground, however, belongs to the actor and translates through subjective perceptions into "decisions" to act which are rather unpredictable in their specifics.

Finally, is this volition fully free will or rational?[6] The answer is probably the same as David Matza (1964) hazarded: a form of soft determinism. If all possible background factors were known and the situation fully analyzable in a linear fashion, the actor's subjective perceptions might be somewhat predictable. Because we do not have such rich information and because the world contains non-linearity, for our purposes the actor's behavior remains unpredictable even if it is deterministic. However, this interpretation does have the advantage of introducing some element of independent choice into the actor's world and explains the chaotic nature of individual decisions.

Incorporating Subjectivity

Comments in an earlier chapter indicated a need to bring subjectivity back into criminology. The question now is how subjectivity is to be incorporated into a chaos-based reality? First, I need to reiterate that individuals make subjective assessments on a daily basis. This is the way humans live; they all perceive the reality around them, interpret it through their shared and unique experiences and ideologies, and then make decisions to act (perhaps a sort of unconscious, soft, rational-choice model). Even quantitative researchers do this when they are not doing research (and, of course, do it in subtle ways when they *are* doing research). Indeed, human subjectivity is so pervasive that it is a wonder that social science has not incorporated it as a staple in all analyses and theories. Second, it should also be clear that subjectivity alone is responsible for some of the chaos of reality. With subjective decisions being made in objectively similar situations, the range of choices begins to appear as chaotic noise in linear social science data. In other words, attempts to predict those decisions are burdened with varying choices that are chaotic. In order to know with accuracy what choices will be made minimally requires an *a priori* knowledge of the subjective framework in which those choices will transpire. This is what one might refer to as background data on the subjects and it is very difficult to come by.

How does subjectivity come into play and what are the sources of this subjectivity? There appear to be three notable sources: (1) the background of the individual contains previous subjective assessments, (2) previous experiences of the subject are reinterpreted subjectively, or

(3) the current situation/environment is interpreted subjectively. First, the background of an individual is a product of biogenetic, environmental, psychological, and sociological factors. That combination contributes to the various decisions that an individual makes throughout life. *Each time* a decision is made, those factors come into play to assist in interpretation of the event and, over time, structure an ideology by which multiple events are interpreted. Thus, a lifetime of subjective reality exists for all humans. This is the subjective background that, across different individuals, results in objective unpredictability of any one individual's choices. To the extent individuals share a large portion of their subjective background (subculture and environment particularly), we might expect greater similarity in regard to the effect of that background in the making of foreground decisions.

Second, the mere existence of a subjective background is insufficient, in and of itself, to affect directly a contemporaneous decision. That background is itself channeled through a subjective assessment. Similar to the process of retrospective interpretation, the background applies only as retrospectively reassessed and subjectively interpreted by the individual. That is, what an individual brings as past baggage is always reinterpreted by the knowledge and ideology of the moment. The subjective background is subjectively reinterpreted to fit with contemporaneous subjective reality. As a consequence, even objective knowledge of an individual's subjective background will not yield accurate prediction because the subjective reinterpretation of that background introduces another chaotic factor.

Third, the remaining source of a subjective interpretation of reality lies in the environment and situation of the moment. If any, this is the realm of subjectivity that analysts normally discuss. The individual's view of environment and situation is, of course, already tempered with experience and background. At the instant of decision, however, a smoothly linear effect does not seem likely. Indeed it is more probable that the individual acts from passions and emotions that color not only the objective reality but also his or her experience and background. Thus, the more highly charged the situation is for the individual, the less likely is the predictability of any behavior. What the individual sees and feels becomes more subjective in such a scenario. Conversely, in unemotional situations we would expect the individual's actions to become more predictable.

These three sources of subjectivity apply directly to individual behavior. The behavior of groups, an aggregate function, is of course a product of the individual choices, but more structured. Because of the potential similarity of background and ideology from which to interpret and the probable commonality of environment and situation, contemporaneous group actions are more likely to have predictable patterns. While this predictability will not be anywhere near perfect, it should be obvious that certain patterns will develop in the data. These patterns are the ones observed in subcultural theories and in virtually all research based on structural or ecological variables. As with virtually all chaotic data, patterns exist and replicate themselves as one moves from the individual case to ever larger aggregates. I suspect that it is the tendency to work with aggregate data that allows social scientists to ignore the presence and effect of subjectivity.

Expressly placing this into a critical-incident perspective, I find that subjectivity obviously increases the chaotic nature of decisions and, therefore, behavior. Building and maintaining a life-shape is partially a series of previous subjective decisions, enhanced at any moment by an individual's awareness of the background those decisions come to represent. The awareness is filtered through subjective reinterpretation. All things being equal, as the slope moves toward criticality, it is this history and its interpretation that assists in determining whether the slope becomes near-critical or not. An individual with a near-critical slope is ready for an instant situation to change the slope to a critical one. The difference in criticality is at least partially governed by the interpretation of the instant situation. If emotion and passion are high, the slope is likely to become critical (or head toward a supercritical stage). If not, the slope can remain in a near-critical stage or even decrease in criticality.

As an example, imagine an individual who has an experiential background of poverty and frustration, perceives that background as being intolerable, and has developed an extroverted personality. Given a situation that can be viewed as a personal challenge and which promises to add to the built-up frustration, such an individual will probably assess the situation as highly damaging and react in an escalated manner.

While this example may sound like common sense, the difficulty in prediction is knowing the subjective sources that the individual will draw upon in making an instant decision to act (and then, of course, there are multiple acts to choose from). At any rate, subjectivity is important in building and maintaining a life-shape and in escalating that shape toward the critical point. Criminology *must* incorporate subjectivity, with or without a critical-incident perspective, or little progress can be made toward understanding action.

CONCLUSION

There are advantages to a dynamic, nonlinear perspective in attempting to understand deviant behavior (any behavior, for that matter). I am not denying that some portions of reality are linear, or nearly so. It simply makes sense to acknowledge the evidence for pervasive nonlinearity that physicists and others have accumulated. The discussion in this chapter has been designed to show how such a nonlinear approach can assist in interpreting the criminological reality we already know.

Existing unit theories, which encompass virtually all of the theories of criminology, are not jettisoned by the concepts developed thus far. The value of any metatheory is that it provides a way of organizing and making sense of the predictions and observations of unit theories. So far, it is clear that structural theories are more likely to benefit from a critical-incident metatheory than are processual theories. Aggregated, time-series data are simply more conducive to locating patterns in chaotic systems than are individual-level data. Should the latter be available in time series with sufficient depth of information, there is no reason why patterns cannot be located there also. Such data are unusual in criminology, however.

The next chapter, the final one, continues the dialog about what criminology ought to be doing.

NOTES

1. By "proximate" I refer to those variables that are closely linked in time with the dependent variable. The most proximate variable would be the last thing that happened to an individual before action took place.

2. I use the term "group-shape" as a reminder that life-shapes are not limited to individuals.

3. There is also the possibility that the individual subjectively interprets the external conditions in a different fashion than an outside observer expects.

4. Yes, Merton systematically used the term "individual" in his explanation of the theory (1938). However, he was following the Parsonian approach (ego and alter) to discussing the collective as if it were an individual.

A reference to an "individual" by Merton was invariably a reference to a constituent of the social collective.

5. In one sense, it makes no difference whether the universe is deterministic or not. A willed choice to behave in response to certain pressures is at once both deterministic and free willed. The pressures force the issue and a rational (or even irrational) choice to behave allows the individual to maintain his or her sense of control. One potential choice, which confounds existing analytical schemes, is to do nothing. Oddly enough, Robert Merton introduced this very concept into his scheme of deviance with his inclusion of conformity as a mode of *deviance*, yet few have seen its value.

6. By the term "rational" I do not mean that an actor engages in a logically-constrained series of thoughts that assess the situation in a cost-benefit manner. Indeed, I assume that the actor's emotional framework and reaction to the situation are at least as important to decision-making as constrained rationality.

REFERENCES

Akers, Ronald L. (1985). *Deviant Behavior: A Social Learning Approach*, 3rd ed. Belmont, CA: Wadsworth.

Bernard, Thomas J. (1987). Testing structural strain theories. *Journal of Research in Crime and Delinquency*, 24:262–280.

Bursik, Robert J., Jr. (1986). Ecological stability and the dynamics of delinquency. Pp. 35–66 in Albert J. Reiss, Jr. and Michael Tonry (eds.) *Communities and Crime. Crime and Justice: A Review of Research*, vol 8. Chicago, IL: University of Chicago Press.

Gottfredson, Michael, and Travis Hirschi (1990). *A General Theory of Crime*. Stanford, CA: Stanford University Press.

Homans, George C. (1964). Bringing men back in. *American Sociological Review* 29: 809–818.

Matza, David (1964). *Delinquency and Drift*. New York, NY: Wiley.

McShane, Marilyn D., and Frank P. Williams III (1985). Anomie theory and marijuana use: Clarifying the issues. *Journal of Crime and Justice* 8, 2: 21–40.

Merton, Robert K. (1938). Social structure and anomie. *American Sociological Review* 3: 672–682.

Osgood, D. Wayne, Janet K. Wilson, Patrick M. O'Malley, Jerald G. Bachman, and Lloyd D. Johnston (1996). Routine activities and individual deviant behavior. *American Sociological Review*, 61:635–655.

Schuerman, Leo, and Solomon Kobrin (1988). Community careers in crime. Pp. 67–100 in Albert J. Reiss, Jr. and Michael Tonry (eds.) *Communities and Crime. Crime and Justice: A Review of Research*, vol 8. Chicago, IL: University of Chicago Press.

Walker, Jeffery T. (1996). Chaos theory and social disorganization: A new paradigm for neighborhood analysis. Paper presented at the annual meeting of the Academy of Criminal Justice Sciences, Las Vegas, NV.

CHAPTER TEN

Conclusions

In case it has not yet become evident, the purposes of this book are best described as an argument for a perspective on reality that offers (1) an appreciation of real-world complexity in theory construction, (2) an interdisciplinary approach to locating important variables in determining behavior, (3) the encouragement of nonlinear, nonproximate conceptions of causality and (4) an understanding of the role of subjectivity in individual behavior. More important than the theoretical approach taken to the metatheory are the implications of new forms of discovering patterns or structure within our data. Systematic conceptions of causality need to be redefined so that non-sequential and nonadditive effects can be located and, ultimately, understood. A new paradigm of interpretation is needed in criminology before these changes can take place.

WHY METATHEORY?

Rather than present a theory of criminal behavior I have chosen to construct a metatheory. This was done for several reasons. First, I believe that criminology is now at the stage where we need new ways to look at old ideas. The fact that we keep looking at old ideas is relatively incontrovertible. Virtually all existing, mainstream theories are plays upon older theory and reuse the basic variables from the first half of this century. While there is nothing wrong with revisiting old ideas, we desperately need to combine them with new ideas.

Second, I believe that virtually all unit theories have grasped some piece of reality. In other words, each one of our existing theories reflects something that rings true in our experiences. But at the same time, I am convinced that those theories are bound by situation, time, and space. That is, they are somewhat idiosyncratic and apply to a special group of people at some contemporaneous moment. Looking back across the past century of theory, I am more and more convinced that this is true. It may be that we do not need more theory right now. Instead, we may need a sense of how to view the theories we have. In short, we need a better grasp on human and social reality. Once we have that, we may even find new ways to use existing theory.

A third reason for choosing metatheory over theory is that it offers a challenge to others to make explicit the assumptions about the world that they are now keeping implicit. It would be quite instructive to hear how the various authors of existing unit theories view reality—and it may be surprising as well. If for no other reason, proposing an orienting perspective is helpful in making us question our assumptions. As a field, we have not done that since the emergence of labeling and conflict theories during the 1960s.

Another reason is that a metatheory allows commentary on method as well as theory. Because metatheories discuss *how* to view a phenomenon, they explicitly propose standards and approaches for measurement. Criminologists have spent long enough in the linear, quantitative paradigm. It is time to question why we believe that numbers are the best way to represent human reality and to extend the way we gather evidence on human decision-making behavior. Indeed, it is time to ask how individual's experiences affect their behavior. And, of course, ways need to be found to measure the answers to that question.

Fifth, because a metatheory incorporates unit theories, it offers the ability to reconcile them. It would be instructive simply to investigate the ways in which existing theories interact with each other. The fact is that they don't all attempt to explain the same thing. Yet our penchant for competition and choosing the "best" theory patently ignores that fact. This is particularly the case for the various generic forms, such as control, learning, strain, conflict, and postmodern theories. Questions to be asked are: How do they differ? What do they have in common? In what ways may they be combined to better represent reality?

Finally, criminology has probably reached the point where integration of theories is a virtual necessity. Those who take the stance that concepts are "owned" and peculiar to "their" theory are failing to recognize the larger picture. While each of the unit theories reflects reality at some time and place, it is clear that each does not reflect all of reality. Further, I do not expect any theorist to have discerned more than a piece of reality; that small effort alone is a major insight of which most of us are not capable. The arguments in earlier chapters suggest that the forces that govern human action are most likely composed of factors from many sources and certainly not just from sociological variables. From this perspective, then, it makes sense to join as many pieces of reality as we can find to see what develops. This joining process is the integration of unit theories.

For these reasons, and more that are evident in earlier discussion, I believe that metatheories are needed now to prod criminologists into asking questions and seeking new ways to view existing answers. I also believe that we have gotten so critical of unit theories that a fresh way of looking at the world would help us see the value in what we already have. The role of these expectations plays an important part in conceptual development.

What Do We Expect of Theories?

It seems to me that social scientists, particularly as critics, expect much more of any theory than we do of reality. This is a rather strange happenstance. Within the context of reality, we are generally happy when most observations match our perceptions. Even this target of "most observations" is deceptive. Humans are universally guilty of using selective and biased observations to structure and make sense of the world about them. The hard fact is that reality is too complex for full comprehension; therefore, not everything corresponds with our selective view of the way things "ought to be." Nonetheless, the way we live our lives suggests that such approximations are adequate. We successfully negotiate and survive most obstacles regardless of the fact that our perception and understanding of the world are inadequate and faulty.

Where theory is concerned, theorists often make claims about reality that seem to require the existence of broad supporting evidence. Although that may be correct, it is more likely that in the creation of the theory some degree of misstatement about reality has taken place. That is, the importance of some variable or causal agent (even if true) has been exaggerated. This is so for the same reasons that selective observation leads us to make generalized statements about phenomena that are not necessarily true. We *make* important those things that we believe are important.

Additionally, the evidence-production methods which most theories rely upon are, historically, continually mistaken about the exact nature of things. Even if the theory is correct, there is some likelihood that any evidence gathered will be incorrect. Such a happenstance is particularly problematic when the approved method used to collect the evidence is at fault, yet reliable. Over time, methodologies come and go and are deemed more or less valid at various historical moments. In the context of their time, however, they tend to rule the understanding of reality. If methodologies can be popular yet substantially incorrect in capturing reality, where are the dismissed theories that we should have resurrected for another test?

Combining both of these problems (exaggeration and misstatement with the fallibility of method), it is possible that unit theories will require supporting evidence that was never necessary or even available to begin with. In any given time period, how true can a theory be? If the answer is it doesn't need to be *all* true, what degree of truth will we accept? Indeed, the (eternal) problem is to define acceptability and then to determine the degree of evidence needed find a theory acceptable. It is possible for a theory to be mostly incorrect and still be useful.

In short, three questions need to be asked before we put any unit theory to test:

1. Given the complexity of reality, do we expect any theory to capture much of it?
2. Is there a limit to the amount of evidence available to support any theory in any historical epoch?
3. Just how much of reality needs to match a theory before it can be determined to be useful?

Potential Critiques of the Metatheory

I foresee two general critiques of the content of this book. First, many will object to the "discursive" style of theorizing and critique. It is not tied directly to empirical theory construction and no hypotheses, propositions, or axioms have been presented for testing. Further, much of the discussion will appear to be commonsense and trite. To save time, I now plead guilty to all of these things.

In defense, though, I must say that none of these potential criticisms are bothersome. Metatheories are not designed for testing— they are expressly constructed as ways to view the world and point to what we should be looking for. Unit theories, constructed under a metatheory, are faced with the task of being measurable and testable. To my mind, that is the harder task and I suppose that I am simply not up to it. The appearance of commonsense observations and trite comments, if they really exist, are perhaps the "empirical reality" of metatheory. If comments ring a bell, belie a shared experience, or sound true on their face, then the picture of reality presented within these pages has some degree of validity.

The second critique is, even if all this were reflective of reality, there is no way to prove it. Such a critique is actually a comment on the present state of methodology and it is true we do not have much in the way of analytical tools for exploring chaotic dynamic systems. There are some modeling programs currently under construction, one at the Santa Fe Institute and one in North Carolina. These, however, will but make some initial forays into complex systems analysis for the social sciences. So, we simply do not yet have the methodology for producing evidence. Those who believe strictly in evidence-derived theory (and reality) will no doubt declare an impasse and return to testing what we already know with the same old tired methodologies. Others, who take the view that conceptualizing can precede evidence (sometimes well before evidence is available), will be ready to move on to investigating possibilities and perhaps even constructing the evidence-producing tools necessary to find those possibilities. I believe that the latter is the more advantageous position, largely because it is the way in which novel ideas are formed.

Making More and Better Use of the Criminological Imagination

At the risk of sounding trite and commonsensical, I want to re-emphasize a major undercurrent that runs throughout this book. Criminology (and other social sciences) needs to see the world as the dynamic, complex reality it is. The elevation of one approach so that it dominates thinking is tantamount to reducing the world to an artificial entity. Of course, that makes "explanation" easier, because artificial entities are more simplistic and easily understood. The social sciences really need to endorse a multiplicity of perspectives and methodologies and then use them all to determine where reality lies. Imagination should be endorsed and cultivated.

If one reads Kuhn's (1970) work, or even simply peruses the development of chaos theory, there appears to be an inescapable conclusion about the history of inventions, new ideas, and breakthroughs. They are mostly likely to happen when someone from outside the field, on the periphery or new to it gets interested in a problem. This occurs because that person comes to the problem with perceptions, training, and methodologies that differ from those dominating the field. In short, they *think differently* from the standard thinking of a discipline. As our disciplines have grown narrower and narrower and quantitative methodology so pervasive, we are in danger of losing the capacity to think differently. Under these circumstances, a breakthrough can become another way to measure a standard variable.

Assuming we have lost at least some degree of creativity, how has this happened and how can we avoid it? While there are many answers to these two questions, I wish to focus on one in particular: organization. As disciplines become more organized and structured, they create restrictions in how their scholars work and think. As scholarly organizations develop and mature, they help guide the scholarship of the discipline. And as scholars within those organizations mature, they become honored for the work they have done. All of these things create latent by-products that constrain imagination. The "approved" methodologies provide subtle inducements to work within them and constrain alternative approaches. Disciplines approach problems in certain ways; for scholars to do otherwise is to invite criticism and, potentially, loss of reputation. Honored professors serve as role models for young, emerging scholars, thus serving as a continued link to dominant approaches of the past. All these things are what postmodernists might refer to as "privileged" modes of discourse. Organization serves many functions, but one should not forget that it also serves to perpetuate itself.

If organization restricts thinking, how may greater creativity occur without dismissing organization? In short, how can one be a divergent criminologist without dismissing criminology as a discipline? In an earlier work (Williams, 1984), that question was answered by encouraging analogous thinking (using non-related phenomena to create analogies of the problem at hand) and true multi-disciplinary graduate education. While those solutions might still be valuable, I want to discuss something entirely different and novel. I want the field to encourage *play*.

No, I don't mean that criminologists should engage in a handy game of tag football. I mean that playful thinking should be encouraged.[1] In an era of information technology, there should be means of offering ideas and building wildly upon them. Use-groups, or list-servers, on the Internet[2] can be developed in much greater number than we currently have and people, in and outside of the field, can engage in discussions with little threat to disciplinary egos. Our graduate students should be rewarded for innovative thinking instead of producing rote repetition of the instructor's favorite lines. All in all, in the name of creativity, it would be wise to take ourselves a bit less seriously.

The Upcoming Century

We are now at the turn of a century. If for no other reason, that fact alone suggests we are at a handy point to reassess where we have been and what we have been doing. The dawn of a new century has historically been a time of exploration and ideas. This is the obvious time for trying something new. Unless I am sorely mistaken, activity and creativity in criminology have been increasing during the decade.[3] Nothing has yet occurred, though, to prompt most criminologists to take seriously the need for change, for advancement, and for new modes of thinking. This book was written in that spirit. If it has no other effect than making some people angry, then its purpose will have been served. Scholars should be thinking people and thinking people do their work better without restraints. This critique and the metatheory presented are roadmaps toward lifting existing restraints. I really do not care if this becomes the roadmap people use or not, but I do want criminologists to become more accomplished mental travelers. Then we can all benefit from a diversity of thought.

Finally, I wish to end by reemphasizing something I have said previously, but which will probably be missed by those who are vested in quantitative criminology. I *support* quantitative methodology—I just don't believe it should dominate our mode of thinking. The use of quantitative methodology is absolutely necessary for the advancement of the discipline. However, qualitative methodology is equally necessary. *All* forms of evidence-gathering tools should be used in our quest for a view of reality. As fixation on a theoretical approach is dangerous to the health of the field, so too is fixation on one form of analysis or method. Thus, the new century of criminology will be, I hope, a diverse mixture of both theory *and* method.

NOTES

1. In a recent discussion with Jeff Ferrell, we hit on the idea of "criminological jazz," a jam session for criminological concepts. The idea was to diverge from the usual panel format at a national conference and simply invite scholars to discuss some of the novel things they had been playing with. The "jam" analogy would bring others into the fray, enlarging and modifying the thoughts to see what develops. This is quintessentially what I mean by the concept of *play*.

2. There already is an Internet use-group: alt.criminology. In addition there are several discussion lists where people of various degrees of training in criminology and criminal justice swap e-mail on a multitude of topics.

3. So many new approaches and theoretical commentaries have been developed during the past ten years that it is difficult to even list them. Those that come to mind include John Hagan's (1989) power-control theory, Terence Thornberry's (1987) interactional theory, Marvin Krohn's (1986) network theory, John Braithwaite's (1989) shaming and reintegration theory, Raymond Paternoster and Lee Iovanni's (1989) modified labeling theory, Bruce Link et al.'s (1989) modified labeling model, Robert Sampson and John Laub's (1993) life-course theory, Michael Gottfredson and Travis Hirschi's (1990) self-control theory, Richard Quinney's (1988) and Harold Pepinsky's (1991) (and both, 1991) peacemaking criminology, Dragan Milovanovic's (1997) postmodern theory, Jock Young's (1992) square of crime, Jack Katz's (1988) subjective theory, Rodney Stark's (1987) deviant place theory, Steven Messner and Richard Rosenfeld's (1994) institutional anomie theory, Robert Agnew's (1992) general strain theory, Glenn Walters and Thomas White's (1989) cognitive theory, Jeff Ferrell's (1993) anarchist theory, Hans Eysenck's (1989) personality theory, James Messerschmidt's (1997) structured-action theory, Lawrence Cohen and Richard Machalek's (1988) evolutionary ecology theory, Harold Grasmick and Robert Bursik's (1990) social deterrence model and many more.

REFERENCES

Agnew, Robert (1992). Foundation for a general strain theory of crime and delinquency. *Criminology* 30: 47–88.

Braithwaite, John (1989). *Crime, Shame, and Reintegration.* Cambridge, UK: Cambridge University Press.

Cohen, Lawrence E., and Richard Machalek (1988). A general theory of expropriative crime: An evolutionary ecological approach. *American Journal of Sociology* 94: 465–501.

Eysenck, Hans J. (1989). Personality and Criminality: a Dispositional Analysis. Pp. 89–110 in William S. Laufer and Freda Adler (eds.) *Advances in Criminological Theory*, vol. 1. New Brunswick, NJ: Transaction.

Ferrell, Jeff (1993). *Crimes of Style: Urban Graffiti and the Politics of Criminality*. New York, NY: Garland.

Gottfredson, Michael, and Travis Hirschi (1990). *A General Theory of Crime*. Stanford, CA: Stanford University Press.

Grasmick, Harold G., and Robert J. Bursik (1990). Conscience, significant others, and rational choice: Extending the deterrence model. *Law and Society Review* 24: 837–862.

Hagan, John (1989). *Structural Criminology*. New Brunswick, NJ: Rutgers University Press.

Katz, Jack (1988). *Seductions of Crime: Moral and Sensual Attractions in Doing Evil*. New York, NY: Basic Books.

Krohn, Marvin D. (1986). The web of conformity: A network approach to the explanation of delinquent behavior. *Social Problems* 33: 581–593.

Kuhn, Thomas (1970). *The Structure of Scientific Revolutions*, 2nd ed. Chicago, IL: University of Chicago Press.

Link, Bruce, Francis T. Cullen, Elmer Struening, Patrick E. Shrout, and Bruce P. Dohrewend (1989). A modified labeling theory approach to mental disorders: An empirical assessment. *American Sociological Review* 54: 400–423.

Messerschmidt, James (1997). *Crime as Structured Action: Gender, Race, Class, and Crime in the Making*. Thousand Oaks, CA: Sage.

Messner, Steven F., and Richard Rosenfeld (1994). *Crime and the American Dream*. Belmont, CA: Wadsworth.

Milovanovic, Dragan (1997). *Postmodern Criminology*. New York, NY: Garland.

Paternoster, Raymond, and Lee Iovanni (1989). The labeling perspective and delinquency: An elaboration of the theory and assessment of the evidence. *Justice Quarterly* 6: 359–394

Pepinsky, Harold E. (1991). *The Geometry of Violence and Democracy*. Bloomington, IN: Indiana University Press.

Pepinsky, Harold E., and Richard Quinney (eds.) (1991). *Criminology as Peacemaking*. Bloomington, IN: Indiana University Press.

Quinney, Richard (1988). Crime, suffering, service: Toward a criminology of peacemaking. *Quest* 1: 66–75.

Sampson, Robert J., and John H. Laub (1993). *Crime in the Making: Pathways and Turning Points Through Life*. Cambridge, MA: Harvard University Press.

Stark, Rodney (1987). Deviant places: A theory of the ecology of crime. *Criminology* 25: 893–909.

Thornberry, Terence P. (1987). Toward an interactional theory of delinquency. *Criminology* 25: 863–891.

Walters, Glenn D., and Thomas W. White (1989). The thinking criminal: A cognitive model of lifestyle criminality. *Criminal Justice Research Bulletin* 4(4): 1–10.

Williams, Frank P., III (1984). The demise of the criminological imagination: A critique of recent criminology. *Justice Quarterly* 1: 91–106.

Young, Jock (1992). Ten points of realism. Pp. 24–68 in Jock Young and Roger Matthews (eds.) *Rethinking Criminology: The Realist Debate*. London, UK: Sage.

Index

CURRENT ISSUES IN CRIMINAL JUSTICE
FRANK P. WILLIAMS III AND MARILYN D. MCSHANE
Series Editors